FIRST
DOWN
TO
TOUCHDOWN

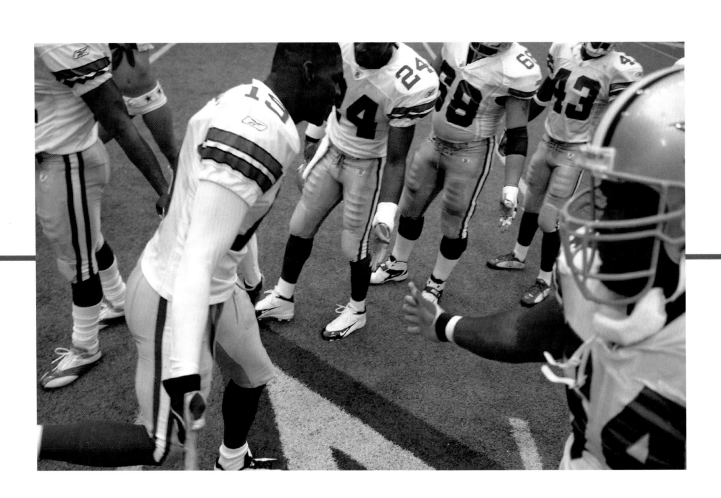

FROM
FIRST
DOWN
TO
TOUCHDOWN

Keyshawn's Keys to Winning in Life

Keyshawn Johnson & James Strom

with Kid Peligro

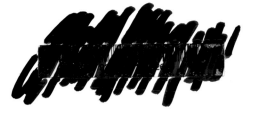

Invisible Cities Press
50 State Street
Montpelier, VT 05602
www.invisiblecitiespress.com

Library of Congress Cataloging-in-Publication Data

Johnson, Keyshawn.
From first down to touchdown : Keyshawn's keys to winning in life /
Keyshawn Johnson and James Strom with Kid Peligro.
p.   cm.
ISBN 1-931229-39-2 (alk. paper)
1. Physical fitness. 2. Conduct of life. I. Strom, James. II. Peligro, Kid. III. Title.
GV481.J67 2004
613.7'1--dc22

2004027030

Anyone practicing the techniques in this book does so at his or her own risk. The authors and the publisher
assume no responsibility for the use or misuse of information contained in this book or for any injuries that
may occur as a result of practicing the techniques contained herein. The illustrations and text are for infor-
mational purposes only. It is imperative to practice these holds and techniques under the strict supervision
of a qualified instructor. Additionally, one should consult a physician before embarking on any demanding
physical activity.

Printed in The United States of America

Photographs appearing on pages ii, viii, 2, 4, 13, 17, 22, 23, 26, and 41 are by James D. Smith
Photographs appearing on pages 9 and 21 are courtesy of USC Athletic Department
All other photographs by Tom Page

Book design by Peter Holm, Sterling Hill Productions

CONTENTS

Plyometrics

Power Series

Fieldwork Exercises

PART THREE: Putting It All Together

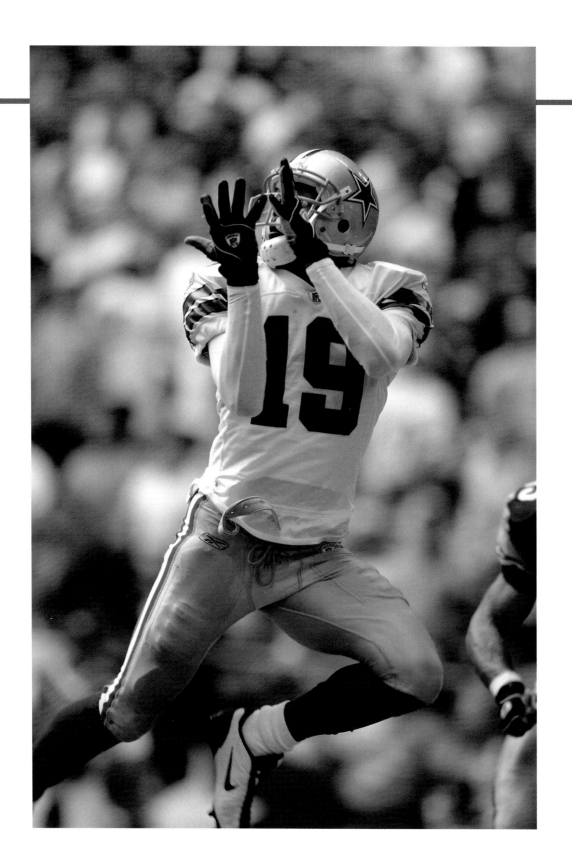

INTRODUCTION

The key to success is to keep growing in all areas of life—mental, emotional, spiritual, as well as physical.

Julius Irving

Over the years you've been watching me on Sundays make the tough catches. Running up the middle with no fear of 200-pound safeties coming at me full speed wanting to take my head off. In my mind, there is only one thought: "Catch the ball! Make it happen!" The consequences are not important to me; it is the task and the result that matter. I get paid a lot of money to catch the ball. I get paid to make things happen! I get paid to win!

Come Sunday, everyone expects me to be on the field, giving it my all on every play, but nobody, I mean nobody, expects more of me than I do! Come Sunday I have to be ready to play. Come Sunday I have to make the catches. Come Sunday I have to win, no excuses!

For me to be able to help my team, I need to be on the field, at the top of my game physically, mentally, and spiritually. People often ask me how I've managed to stay so durable over my football career. In an era when wide receivers are hung out for abuse like piñatas at a birthday party, I'm in there day in and day out, making my catches, scoring my points, hitting my blocks, still running the inside routes. Season after season, I'm in for all sixteen games.

My first answer when people ask me about this is conditioning. To play wide receiver into your thirties in the NFL, you need to stay as strong and quick as possible. I was lucky to have hooked up at USC with a truly extraordinary trainer, James Strom. James and I became good buddies, and he's kept giving me training advice throughout my pro career. It's helped keep me one step ahead of the competition—and it's helped me get back up after those skull-rattling hits.

Enough fans have asked me about this training regimen that I decided to put it down in a book. You have it all here—what I believe is the best general conditioning program you'll find anywhere. It's an excellent workout for everyone, whether you spend ten hours a day in an office or a truck. But it's especially good for anyone who needs speed, strength, and stamina to do their job or their hobby.

But after James and I had put down our workout program, I got to thinking about what has really allowed me to achieve so much in my career. Sure, the physical part of it is essential, but it's nothing without the right mental attitude. If I hadn't believed in myself and developed mental habits that got me through some tough times, I never would have made it to a place where I had my own trainer, that's for sure!

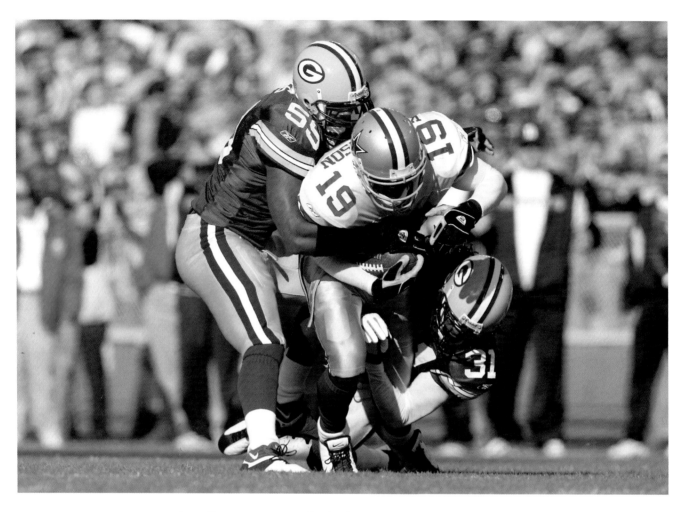

I see a lot of guys—some at the highest levels of competition—who are in great physical shape, but somehow never quite pull their careers and personal lives together because they don't have the mental toughness. So I didn't want to create a book that was just going to make more hard-bodies who melt under pressure. I want this to be a fitness book that can give readers the mental strength to deal with whatever they are going to face and overcome any obstacles that they have to contend with and still reach and work and become the best, regardless of how people try to deter them. That's why I wrote the first part of this book—to let you in on the secrets that have served me so well in keeping my *mind* as fit as my body.

These practices have also allowed me to overcome some daunting obstacles in my life. Poverty, homelessness, crime, jail—I had it all thrown at me before I could even drive. Even fame can be an obstacle, especially because it seems to make happiness that much harder to achieve. Many people make it difficult on themselves to find happiness; they think they must do something magical to achieve it, when really you just have to dig and find happiness within yourself. But fame sometimes means you have to dig all the deeper. Because I've experienced both ends of the spectrum—crushing disappointment and soaring success—I've learned a thing or two about keeping an even keel and finding happiness within.

The passion that you have for life, the desire to be great, is what will serve you best. I always knew what a failure looked like and more than anything I didn't want to be a failure. In my view, spiritual and mental strengths are keys to succeeding in life. If you are true to yourself and your spirit, demand a lot of yourself, have goals and pursue them and, most of all, believe in yourself, there is no obstacle too big to overcome and there is NOTHING YOU CAN'T ACHIEVE!

In Part One of this book I'll give you the keys to becoming mentally and spiritually stronger, to overcoming any obstacle in your path. In Part Two, within the workouts, I'll give you a little reminder of something you can think about or try to put into practice that day. Like anything else, successful mental attitude is a practice that happens once you've internalized it long enough to make it a habit. Habits are automatic; they don't require any extra effort from us.

The most important habit is that of desire. You need to wake up every morning with a burning desire to do something. You need to desire to accomplish something and pursue it with your all. Focus on the objective, the reason for it and the rewards that will come from success. The feeling of accomplishment, the feeling that YOU DID IT! With success, material rewards will follow, but money can't be your goal. If you worry about money, you lose focus. Find what you love to do in life, and everything else will fall into place!

I hope you use this book to get started on a life as successful and fulfilling as mine has been. I know you have everything you need to make this happen—it's just a matter of putting it into play.

Sundays are my days to perform, but my effort and preparation must go in every day. Come Sunday I am ready; come Sunday you will be ready! Everyday in your life is like Sunday in the NFL. I am not into losing and neither are you. Don't hold back, go and BECOME A CHAMPION!

Keyshawn

The fight is won or lost far away from witnesses –
behind the lines, in the gym, and out there on the road,
long before I dance under those lights.

MUHAMMAD ALI

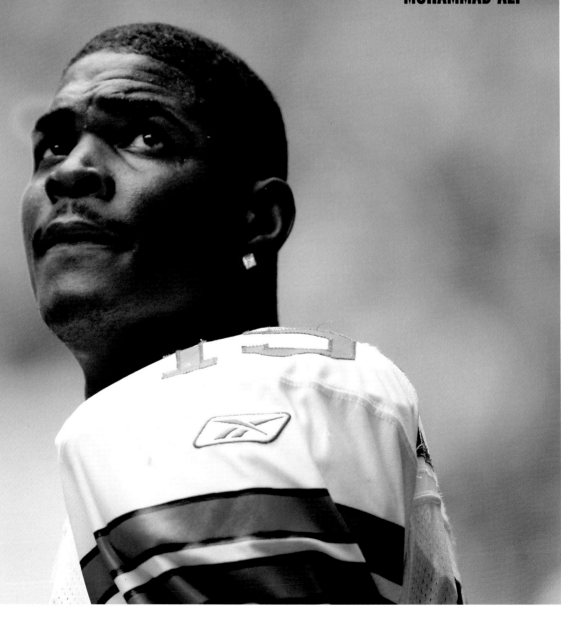

KEYSHAWN'S KEYS TO SUCCESS

1. Believe in Yourself

If my mind can conceive it, and my heart can believe it, I know I can achieve it.

Reverend Jesse Jackson

The first step on your road to success is believing in yourself. If you don't believe you are capable of doing great things, how can you expect anyone else to believe it? You have all the tools you need to be successful at anything you do, right between your ears and inside your chest. With intelligence and heart you can achieve anything you want. I did! I grew up in real, serious poverty in South Central Los Angeles—one of the worst neighborhoods in the country. For a while, when I was ten and eleven, my mother and I were homeless. We lived in our car!

I didn't have a whole lot of prospects for success, but I believed in myself, and that made the difference. I just knew that I didn't want to live under those conditions anymore for any amount of time, and I took matters into my own hands to make sure I didn't. Unfortunately, I had no mentor or guidance, so like a lot of other kids in similar situations, I chose the wrong means, stealing and later dealing drugs. By age twelve, I was providing a home and food for my mother and myself. I don't encourage anyone to take the path I took, but until you walk in a man's shoes you cannot know what drove him to do something.

I did wrong and because of it I had to attend youth camp, but thanks to a guard there named Murphy Ruffin, who gave me the right support and direction, I was able to find the right road and proceed on my path to success. Murphy helped me stay strong and focused, but even with his help it was still up to me to straighten my ways. I had to believe in myself, I had to believe that I could do the things that are necessary in this society to succeed.

I went back to school and began to focus on my athletic career as my way out of the situation I was in. I knew that I didn't have the high-school grades to play ball for a major program. I had to find another way to attract the attention of the colleges. My old coach from Dorsey High, Coach Holmes, told me to come to his new school, West L.A. College, and get my grades up and play. I understood that I had to correct the past and that West L.A. was going to give me the chance to do that. I went there and, after a few more situations and a lot of effort, I was able to get my grades up, catch the attention of the big schools, and was finally able to transfer to USC and Coach Robinson and start to live my dream. It wasn't without trials, but I did it!

Many times in life you will face similar challenges. There are many turning points in life and every decision that you make at that point will affect the rest of your life. No one can be sure at all times of making the right decisions, but no matter what path you take and where life points you to, one of the most important things you can do is have unwavering faith in yourself and your ability to sort things out and persevere in your pursuit of success and happiness. And I say success and happiness because I don't believe you can have one without the other. You have to be happy to be successful and you have to be successful to be truly happy.

Now what is success? It is different for different people. For me, success has meant becoming a top player in the National Football League, graduating from USC, winning the Super Bowl, being able to provide for my mother and my family, and being a good father and a good family man. That last one is a big one for me. When you are raised right on the streets you really don't see a lot of good father figures. I grew up without a father, so I know how tough that is.

Success to you can come in many forms. The first steps in the path to success are very important because, like many things in life, you have to learn to be successful. Success is the result of doing the right thing at the right time and employing all your tools and energies to accomplish the task at hand.

Your road to success begins with little things. Doing well in school, for instance, will teach you how to succeed in smaller projects. In every task you accept, whether it is in school or in real life, you should aim at performing above everyone's expectations.

> The first time I met Keyshawn he was a recruit at USC. When we are trying to recruit kids to come to USC, we give them a pitch. Key walked in and was introduced to me. I started to walk him around the weight room, and he stopped me and said, "Hey, I'm coming here; you don't have to sell me on this. I am going to be the next star coming out of USC." I vividly remember how confident he was. Most young people that come through there are pretty wide-eyed and don't say much and just listen to you and walk out. Keyshawn was special from the first contact. He wasn't overly confident and he wasn't afraid. He was on a mission!
>
> **James Strom**

When things get tough and it looks like you can't do it, remember to believe in yourself and also in the fact that no matter what, things will get resolved one way or another. They may not get resolved the way you want them to, but they will get resolved, and life will move forward. The secret then is to believe in yourself and make every possible effort to direct the results toward what you want.

> Somehow I can't believe that there are any heights that can't be scaled by a man who knows the secrets of making dreams come true. This special secret, it seems to me, can be summarized in four Cs. They are curiosity, confidence, courage, and constancy, and the greatest of all is confidence. When you believe in a thing, believe in it all the way, implicitly and unquestionably.
>
> **Walt Disney**

2. Don't Settle for Less

In order to succeed, your desire for success should be greater than your fear of failure.

Bill Cosby

Many times in life, whether out of convenience, fear, laziness, or because we are afraid of change, we will accept a situation that is not good for us. You cannot do that. If you settle for mediocrity, you will always be mediocre. There are people and situations that bring out the best in you and allow you to perform to the level that you are capable of. You need to seek these people and situations out. Certain people have helped my life tremendously over the years, people like Murphy Ruffin, John Robinson, and Bill Parcells. Because they respect people and care for people, these men have been influential in many lives, including mine. They challenged me to do better and to want more.

We all deserve the best, but many times we settle for less. Had I settled for less I would have probably stayed in South Central L.A., graduated from junior college, and gotten a regular job, but I knew there was more for me in life. There was and still is a fire inside of me that makes me go forward and reach for more. Had I settled for less I probably would have stayed with the New York Jets and I wouldn't have won the Super Bowl! And I wouldn't now be with the Dallas Cowboys.

If you don't look after yourself and demand more for yourself, who else will? If you settle for less, you will never really know what you are capable of. And it is up to you to take care of yourself, because no one is more interested in your well-being and success than you. Mentors are important, but do not put the burden on others to guide you or prod you into higher conquests; it is up to you and you alone to know where you need to go and what is best for you.

Whenever you find yourself in a new situation, analyze if it is good or bad for you. A good situation, be it in life, school, work or family, will help you grow as a person and blossom in the field; a bad situation will cause you to wither. Avoid those at all costs!

Many times in my life I've made the conscious decision not to settle for the status quo. It has to be a conscious decision, a way of forcing your will upon circumstance, because it can be very easy *not* to change. I could have settled for a life of stealing on the streets of L.A.—but I didn't. I made myself make the extra effort to get out, even though it meant more work. I could have settled for playing ball at the junior college level and being a local star—but I didn't. Could have played for USC and not worried about proving to the scouts that I had the speed to play in the pros. Could have spent my whole career with the Jets, cashing my paychecks, making my catches, and not caring whether the team excelled or not. Because I wouldn't settle for less, the Jets improved and so did I.

You get the picture. To get the most out of life, you have to keep your fire, to keep striving to achieve the next level. This won't always be easy; sometimes I've made waves because of my desire to push myself and my teammates. You'd be amazed how at every level, in any field, there are plenty of people who won't like the idea of pushing too hard. People have a lot invested in their own comfort. That's not me. I've never been too comfortable with my own comfort—and you shouldn't be, either! Don't get too comfortable. Don't settle. Keep pushing!

Twenty years from now you will be more disappointed by the things that you didn't do than by the ones you did do. So throw off the bowlines. Sail away from the safe harbor. Catch the trade winds in your sails. Explore. Dream. Discover.
Mark Twain

3. Demand a Lot from Yourself

The quality of a person's life is in direct proportion to their commitment to excellence, regardless of their chosen field of endeavor.
Vince Lombardi

Obviously, If you aren't going to settle for any less than you deserve, then you'd better demand a lot from yourself! Success and happiness are there for you and me, but nothing good in life comes easy. Besides, if it came easy it wouldn't feel half as good.

I have very high expectations for myself and everyone around me. A lot of people want to lower everybody's expectations and goals, so that they don't have to work as hard to be able to say they succeeded. That's a cop-out. If you don't have high expectations and don't demand a lot from yourself, you will never realize your full potential. Look at the time I was with the Jets. We were a lousy team, and it's no fun to play on a lousy team. It becomes tempting to give up, to mail it in. But I was coming from USC, a winning tradition, Cotton Bowl and Rose Bowl winner, and I never liked losing so I made sure I still played my heart out every game. It wasn't going to get us to the playoffs, but it made a big difference to me. I kept demanding more from myself than just about anyone around me, and eventually the results came. We became a playoff club, and I achieved lots of personal success as well.

You can't look to others for your internal motivation. Later in my career I found myself in a situation where I was not in a friendly environment, but I just continued to work at it, didn't stop, didn't stop short of anything, just continued to hammer away at things. I just ran my routes and trained as hard as ever, and eventually things turned. My experience is that they always do.

If you are going to want more, you need to expect more from yourself.

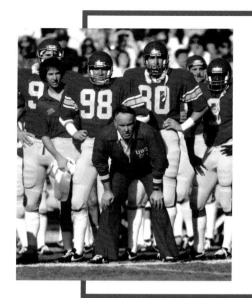

Keyshawn has a great passion for playing. That is probably his greatest characteristic. He can generate that passion for anything he is doing. I recall one practice in particular. In junior college the pace hadn't been as intense as USC, so he ran and we kept yelling for him to run faster and harder and by the end of practice he was just one total body cramp and we had to carry him off the field because he was going to bust his ass till he died. He learned very quickly and would stay out after practice. He just had in his mind the ambition that he was going to succeed, and he would do anything he could to succeed. It was really a pleasure to coach him.

Coach John Robinson

And you need to do this in everything you do, because you need to train yourself to expect more. This is not just a turn-on and turn-off thing. This needs to be your attitude 100 percent of the time. In a word: COMMITMENT! Commitment to yourself and the others around you. The week before the Superbowl I broke a finger on my right hand. One of the coaches asked me if I was going to be able to play. I told him: "I'm playing! I don't care if I can't catch. I'll play special teams if I have to, but I'm playing!"

> There's always the motivation of wanting to win. Everybody has that. But a champion needs, in his attitude, a motivation above and beyond winning.
>
> **Pat Riley**

4. Don't Worry

> There is nothing that wastes the body like worry.
> **Gandhi**

Even if we are good at setting our standards high and pushing ourselves, our minds can sidetrack us. Sometimes we let our emotions distract us from the path to our dream. Other times we allow ourselves to worry about things instead of focusing on the actions we need to take to succeed. Worry is one of the most destructive behaviors, because it almost always involves wasting energy on the unknown, on things we can't control. Don't waste your time and energy worrying about something; *do* something about it instead!

People sometimes ask me how I handle the pressure of being a star in the NFL. You call that pressure? Gimme a break. Pressure is having to worry about scoring some money to feed yourself and your mom. Pressure is dodging bullets in South Central L.A. I get paid a lot of money to play a game. That's not pressure.

When athletes do feel pressure, it's because they've started worrying about other people's expectations for them, or they've taken responsibility for their entire team. That's trouble. Focus on yourself, do what you need to do, and you'll be fine. I know what I have to do, and I do it. Make the blocks, hold on to the pass, juke the cornerback for six points. And inspire my teammates as much as I can. That's all within my control. A lot of other stuff isn't, so I don't worry about it. Everything is going to be resolved one way or another no matter what! The key is to stay in the here-and-now, to apply yourself fully to the task at hand, and do what you can do to make things happen.

A related and important secret to success is to remember that you can only do one thing at a time. Sometimes we let other things in our life enter our mind at a time when we should be focusing on the goal ahead. Extraneous thoughts and events—a family situation, a contract negotiation, a situation at work, or whatever—can take away our energy and focus. When outside things try to affect you, you need to develop a way of blocking them out. To do this, I completely immerse myself in what I am doing. This takes practice. When a distracting thought comes into your head, refocus on a detail of the event at hand. Squeeze that extraneous thought right out of your head by concentrating so intensely on the here-and-now!

When the NCAA came after Keyshawn, they came after him HARD! An hour before practice, four or five guys would sit him in a room and drill him, trying to get him to say certain things, but then of course there was nothing for him to say. After that he'd go to the locker room, get taped and come out. We'd be stretched and warmed up and practicing already and Key would come jogging out on the field as if nothing had happened. He was able to focus and put it away. That was a major distraction that probably would get most players down, but Key would go out and catch fourteen footballs during the game. Something about him allows him to battle these hurdles along the way and not only not get distracted and go in the tank, but actually always come out ahead.

James Strom

Many times in life we worry about missed opportunities, but opportunities occur all the time. Having missed one frees you up to take advantage of the next one. Don't worry about having missed the starting gun, because the starting gun goes off every day when you wake up!

How do you stop worrying? First of all you need to start telling yourself not to worry about things. The mind has immense power; if you allow it to control your actions in a negative way, you will freeze. Learn the difference between worrying and planning. There's nothing wrong with planning for the future—with thinking things through, anticipating the possibilities, and being prepared to act on them. Worrying is when you obsess on the future (or, worse, the past) and work it over again and again in your mind uncontrollably without looking for a solution.

One useful technique is to mentally follow a situation through to the worst possible end. First ask yourself: "What is the worst thing that could happen from this?" Answer it honestly and then begin to develop a plan for the worst case, and if the worst comes you already have a ready response. This way you won't be caught by surprise.

Once you have the worst possible scenario resolved, you can relax. There is nothing else to worry about. You can begin to concentrate your efforts on making sure the situation works out as well for you as possible. Plan for the worst but expect the best!

Another great way to control your worries is to look back at similar experiences and examine what went on before and how it turned out. Did you worry about the situation? Did it help? What was the end result? What could you have done to encourage a better result? By focusing on something in the past you will be able to analyze the problem or task with less emotion (because it has already been determined) and find solutions and paths for your current situation.

> **Do you remember the things you were worrying about a year ago? How did they work out? Didn't you waste a lot of fruitless energy on account of most of them? Didn't most of them turn out all right after all?**
> **Dale Carnegie**

5. Don't Let Others Tell You What You Can or Can't Do

> **I am always doing things I can't do; that's how I get to do them.**
> **Pablo Picasso**

Life is all about choices—*your* choices. One things is for sure: if you allow others to tell you what you can or can't be, or what you can or can't achieve, you leave the control of your life to others. You accept their vision and limitations as yours. The only one who can tell you what you are capable of should be you.

We can even make our own limits. The mind is the most powerful force there is. If you tell yourself you can't do something, you certainly will not be able to do it. Learn to harness the power of your own mind, believe in yourself, and tell yourself you CAN DO! You will be able to accomplish amazing things when you believe in yourself and allow yourself to excel.

All our lives people tell us what we can't do. All my life people said, "You can't!" Even after I became a star at USC, even after I was MVP of the Cotton Bowl my junior year and MVP of the Rose Bowl my senior year, people were *still* saying I couldn't make it in the pros. They admitted I had good hands and a nose for the ball, but they said there was a speed problem. No matter who you are or what level you achieve, some people

All the scouts doubted that Keyshawn had the breakaway speed to make it in the NFL. So we really worked on his speed, his 40-yard-dash time. We had a pro day at USC when all the scouts came to check the players' time, weight, and so on. They came to watch Keyshawn run. It was a zoo. Because I was the head strength coach I had to meet in an auditorium with all the scouts and NFL head coaches that were interested in drafting Keyshawn. They asked me character questions, physical questions, how strong, how fast, does he miss workouts? And my answer to all the questions was: "This guy is amazing. He does whatever it takes. He shows up on Sundays to train, Saturdays to train. Whenever I want him, he's there." So he ran his 40's and blew everybody away. There were a hundred scouts standing at the finish line timing Key, and he ran great. Right then is when we knew he was going to be the first pick of the draft

James Strom

will look for reasons to go after you and tell you "you can't", just because they themselves can't.

Anyway, they had a pro day at USC. All the NFL scouts come to weigh me, time me, poke me, whatever. If I'd believed the things I was hearing about myself, I might not have performed so well that day. But I didn't care what anyone else said. I knew the speed was there—or that I could *make* it be there. I trained hard with James on my forty-yard dash. When the time came, I ran great.

6. Stay Focused on Your Dream

The future belongs to those who prepare for it today.
Malcolm X

It is always important to remain focused on your dream! Along the way there are many distractions that will try to take away your focus. Friends may try to derail you from your ultimate goal, or you may lose focus for many other reasons, personal difficulties, bad luck, illness, stress, whatever. But it is important to remain focused on the dream. Always remind yourself what you ultimately want to achieve and you will find it much easier to stay on course.

Many people are afraid of change. You see this in groups of friends who want to keep everyone at the same level, actually discouraging any of their peers from excelling. If one starts to emerge as a standout in anything, then it shows the others' inadequacies and it takes away their excuses for being mediocre. Don't let your peers or friends hinder your progress toward your dream.

Other times your friends may try to sway you to their "way of success."

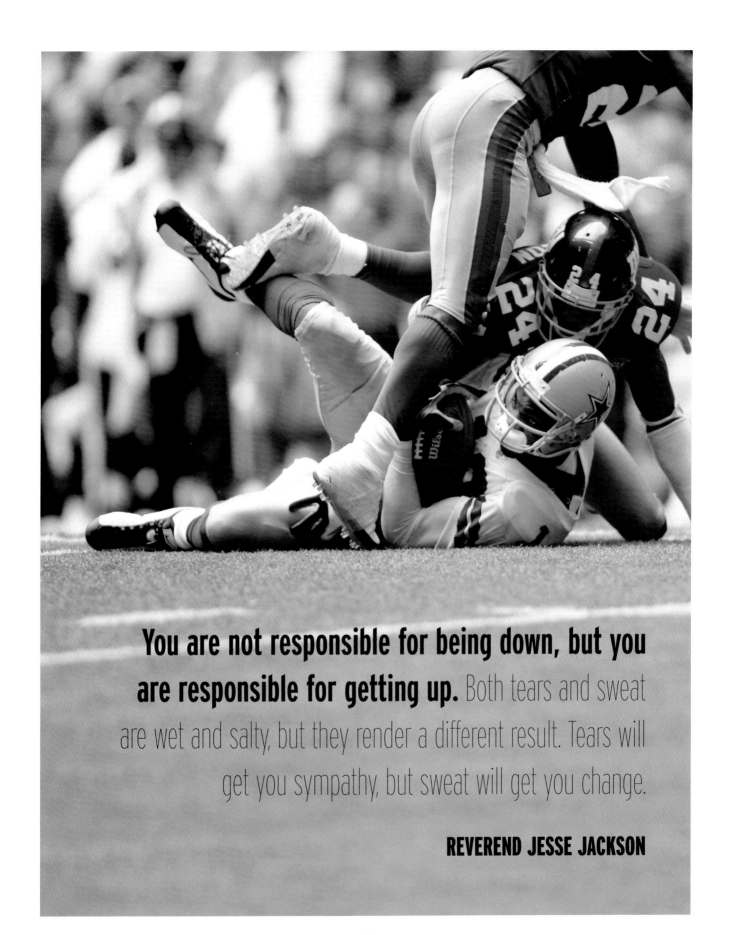

You are not responsible for being down, but you are responsible for getting up. Both tears and sweat are wet and salty, but they render a different result. Tears will get you sympathy, but sweat will get you change.

REVEREND JESSE JACKSON

I've certainly struggled with that. In my youth, I was involved with several illegal activities. I stole bikes, scalped tickets, and even sold drugs to survive when I was homeless. For me it was just business; it was survival. When I was nine or ten I used to wait for the USC football team bus to pull up at games. Coach Robinson would get off first, and I always asked him for extra tickets. He took a liking to me and often gave me a few. Which, of course, I scalped immediately. Sure, I'd have loved to go to the game, but food and rent came first! Coach Robinson asked me about this years later, when I was on the USC team. "Hey coach," I said, " I was a money guy even then!" My methods may have been unorthodox, but even then I had both eyes locked on the prize!

Keep the dream alive. That's one thing you've got to realize: someday the dream will come true, no matter what anyone says. To achieve your dreams, you have to have goals and accept nothing less than those. The key to reaching your dreams is to set big goals, but to have smaller goals and steps that you can reach along the way to keep you fired up and focused. Goal setting is tricky. You need to learn to set your goals so that they challenge you, but you still are able to reach them. You don't want to set them so low that you can reach them without any effort. But if you set them so high that you never reach them, then that won't work for you, either. For instance, you can be in high school and set yourself the goal of becoming a millionaire. That isn't a problem, but you need to realize that the road to being a millionaire involves many other smaller goals and steps that you have to achieve first. Set yourself goals that are neither too easy nor too discouraging and progressively increase the tasks until you achieve your ultimate goal.

Coach Robinson at USC was great at this. He had regular goals for all his players. Everyone knew what they had to do and how they had to perform in order to satisfy their goals and help the team win. I was always focused on a goal and a reward.

Like winning, reaching your goals is a learned experience. The more you set and reach higher and higher goals, the more confidence you will have. You also should have a reward for each goal you achieve. That teaches your mind that the goal is not meaningless; there is an incentive for the accomplishment. As your goals get bigger, your rewards should get bigger as well. But keep things in perspective! Don't give yourself a Ferrari for doing your homework.

> I motivated Keyshawn by saying, "If you do what I ask you to do, I am going to throw you the ball. I am going to use you. We had a goal for him that he'd get a hundred catches each year, and I think on both years he got it. He used to stand behind me in the sidelines and he would say in a low voice, 'Throw the ball to Keyshawn.' He'd whisper in my ear, 'Throw the ball to Keyshawn.' That was always kind of funny. And I wasn't dumb—I was going to throw him the ball!"
>
> **Coach John Robinson**

Another thing to watch out for is setting smaller goals that get in the way of your ultimate goals. For instance, as a wide receiver, my ultimate goal is to have my team win the Super Bowl. I have smaller goals—catching 100 passes a year, scoring ten touchdowns, or whatever—but these only help keep me on course for the big prize, and can be abandoned if necessary. For example, in college I had a long streak of games in which I'd caught passes for at least a hundred yards. In my next game, the other team told me ahead of time that they were going to shut me down. Whatever, I said to myself, so long as we win. That's the whole point. As long as we win I couldn't care less. It's the scoreboard at the end of the day that matters. You might hold me to two yards, and you worked your damnedest to hold me to two yards, you almost killed yourself holding me to two yards, and we still won. Because you paid so much attention to me that you opened up all sorts of other opportunities for us. I contributed to the win in that sense. Football is a team sport. I like setting personal goals for myself, but I don't let them get in the way of the team goals.

> I have coached a lot of great players at USC and the Rams, but Keyshawn is on my all-time team. I'd put him right there with Marcus Allen and Ronnie Lott and those people that just brought something extra to the game.
>
> **Coach John Robinson**

Concentrate on your objective and do not let others distract you from it. Do not worry about what everyone else is doing—though sometimes it helps to use them as incentives to excel. For instance, I don't worry about what other receivers are doing in the league, but I use them as challenges. I try to end up with more receptions than anyone else in the league, or fewer fumbles. But again, we are talking about a team sport. I only use these ways of inspiring myself if it affects my team in a positive way.

> If you're bored with life—you don't get up every morning with a burning desire to do things—then you don't have enough goals.
> **Lou Holtz**

7. Learn from Your Setbacks, Then Move Forward

> If you're trying to achieve, there will be roadblocks. I've had them; everybody has had them. But obstacles don't have to stop you. If you run into a wall, don't turn around and give up. Figure out how to climb it, go through it, or work around it.
> **Michael Jordan**

You have to keep trying even when you fail. *Especially* when you fail. If you fail, you need to get back up and try again and again. Look at me. Many times in my life I've been dealt some pretty severe setbacks. I had several chances of giving up, but always stayed strong and persevered. If I complained about my bad luck or lack of luck, all I would be doing is wasting precious energy on nothing. No one ever succeeded because they complained and no one has ever won because they felt sorry for themselves. Remember, at age nine I was homeless, living in a car with my mother, but I didn't complain and, most of all, I didn't quit!

Quitting is a cop-out. It is the easy way out. "I quit!" There, end of problem. But as the saying goes, quitters don't win and winners don't quit! Quitting is for losers and you and I are not losers. WE ARE WINNERS! Winners use their setbacks and life's hurdles and difficulties as challenges and springboards for success.

When I was deactivated by Tampa in 2003, I could have just shut down. They were literally telling me I couldn't play football! Rather than get down about it, I decided to use it as an opportunity to stretch myself, to try something new. I got a contract with Fox NFL Football, and a week after being deactivated I was sitting on a set with Terry Bradshaw and Howie Long analyzing football. It turned out to be a great experience.

This attitude will change the way you think about risk. Many people fail to achieve simply because they do not want to fail. They don't want to look bad doing something. If you are not willing to take risks, you are not going to excel, because every great accomplishment runs parallel to great failure! But as I've said, failure is just the pit stop on the road to success. Do not be paralyzed by fear of failure, but rather live for the excitement of victory. Dare to take risks without fearing failure!

When you do have a setback or a loss, you need to use that as a motivation to do better the next time. Life is made of peaks and valleys. One of the keys to success is not letting the valleys get you down and taking advantage of the peaks. As you progress in your process of winning, your valleys will become shallower and less frequent and your peaks will be higher and last longer. By learning from your mistakes and forging ahead with your beliefs and full effort, your path to success will always head upward. In time even the valleys will seem more like plateaus than pits.

Also, after every valley there is an even higher peak, so learn to accept and even "like" the valleys, because they are an essential prelude of good things to come. With this kind of mental frame everything in life will be positive and you will be able to think clearly and deal with any situation you are faced with. A setback is a learning experience that gives you an opportunity to grow. Successful people accept and even appreciate the challenges and the falls, knowing they will come out of them wiser and stronger and better able to deal with similar situations in the future.

Now let's be honest. I prefer to win. Give me a choice between winning and losing, I'm going to take winning every time. Who wouldn't? Winning excites me. But, just as with losing, it is important not to dwell on it. When we win a game I say to myself, "You know what, we won a

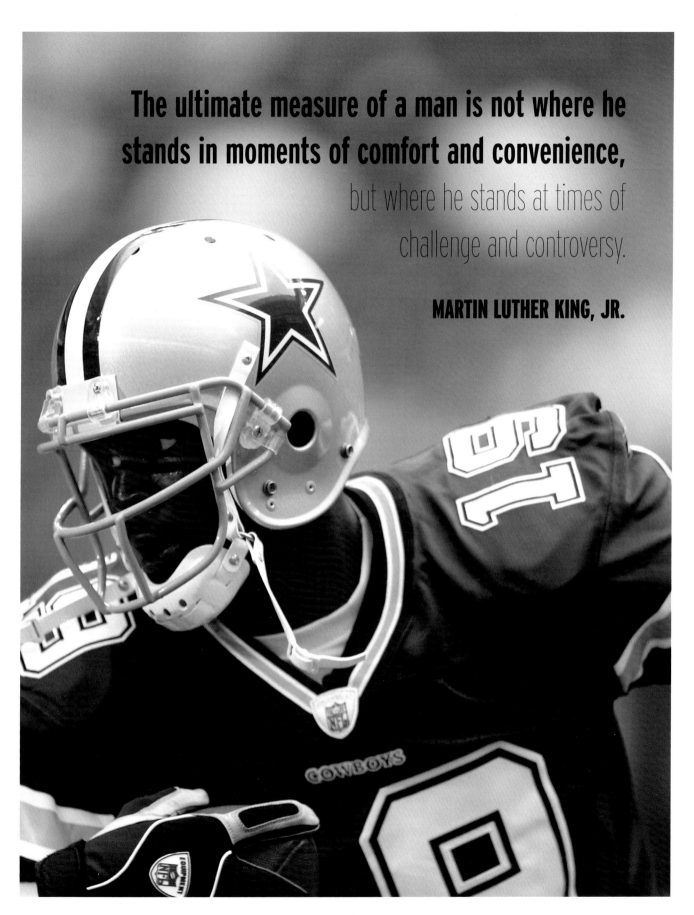

The ultimate measure of a man is not where he stands in moments of comfort and convenience, but where he stands at times of challenge and controversy.

MARTIN LUTHER KING, JR.

football game. Now turn the page." Typically when we win a game I move forward. When we lose it sits with me like a bad steak in my stomach—all the more reason to reexamine what went wrong, why it went wrong, and what I am going to do to correct it and improve and make sure it won't happen again. Then I move on. Either way, you have to keep moving on.

What happens when you don't move on? When you feel bad about the failure or setback and dwell on it aimlessly for days? When you have thoughts like, "Why do things like this always happen to me?" or "I never win anyway." People that react this way to setbacks in life, whether in sports, personal life, or business, set themselves up emotionally and mentally for another failure in the future.

While I don't look for losses as a way to grow, losses are a great motivator to me. You learn more from losing than from winning. Still, I certainly don't want to become a sage by losing frequently, so what I do in case of a loss is to thoroughly examine the events that led to the loss. I analyze everything that I did before the losing day and I also check my preparation for the event. I look back at other failures or setbacks and see if they had anything in common. Was I too cocky thinking that I had the project or the game in hand? Did I underestimate my opponent? Was I prepared? To win consistently in sports, as in life, you always have to go into the "event" knowing that you are at your best. When I go into a game, I always do everything physically, emotionally, and mentally possible to be totally prepared and know that I am there at my best. I know that it all depends on me doing what I do best anyway. I do not have to be thinking, "I should have lifted weights a little more, I am not at the top of my condition," or "I hope they don't throw the ball to me today because I didn't get a chance to practice my catches this week!" If you go into a game thinking about the things you should have done better and that you are not fully prepared for your mission, chances are you will fail.

8. Winning Is an Attitude

"If you want to take your mission in life to the next level, if you're stuck and you don't know how to rise, don't look outside yourself. Look inside. Don't let your fears keep you mired in the crowd. Abolish your fears and raise your commitment level to the point of no return, and I guarantee you that the Champion Within will burst forth to propel you toward victory."

Bruce Jenner

Winning is an acquired technique and a learning process much like anything else. It is also an attitude. Losers begin to lose, and look for excuses to lose, a long time before the battle is played out. Losers can turn a certain victory into a collapsing defeat simply because over the years they have learned to lose! They feel comfortable losing, they understand losing and actually subconsciously sabotage their own efforts. The loser has no responsibility and no new demands. Losing is easy.

Winners are different. They always look for ways, even in the face of huge odds against them, to win and accomplish their tasks. Winners prepare for the win and look forward to the challenge and are willing to do what it takes to put themselves in a position to win. They don't look for excuses, and don't look at previous setbacks as evidence that they will fail. If winners are down by 21 points in the fourth quarter, they are thinking, "How can I get a touchdown to get back in this thing?" Winners are always expecting to win, while losers are always expecting to lose.

Winning is a process just like anything else. Often you'll see a person who has been competing in some field for some time but, despite plenty of talent, has not won anything simply because they have not experienced the taste of victory. They have come close, but they haven't yet learned to master the art of winning. Maybe they are nervous, maybe inexperienced, or maybe they do not yet understand the amount of effort that it takes to win. One way to overcome that and to learn the winning ways is to compete often and get used to the situations. With enough repetition you will become comfortable, less nervous, and be able to perform to your best level.

If you have a problem with winning, try learning the winning habit in smaller, simpler things. Look for less difficult situations that will give you a winning experience. Memorize how it felt to win! Were you nervous? How did you control the nervousness? How did you manage to achieve success? Then try to use the same approach in more complicated or difficult situations. Visualize yourself winning! Play the situation in your mind and try to anticipate the setbacks or problems that can come, and then visualize yourself solving them and succeeding! See yourself at the end of the process, lifting the trophy or taking the victory lap.

Winning is a habit. Unfortunately, so is losing.
Vince Lombardi

9. Don't Forget Who You Are

To be yourself in a world that is constantly trying to make you something else is the greatest accomplishment.
Ralph Waldo Emerson

As you become successful, things may change around you. You begin to see the results of all your effort and your life begins to flourish. Your status improves and your personal satisfaction increases, but with that other problems may arise. It is not uncommon for people, once they realize their dreams or reach their goals, not to be equipped to handle the success. They stop being themselves and stop doing the things that led them to success. They lose sight of what is important to them and become a ship without a rudder, drifting without a set of values.

I certainly ran that risk. I went from being a poor kid in L.A. to being a star with the New York Jets, playing before packed stadiums, making insane money, and enduring the microscope of the New York media. I was lucky because I had been a ball boy at USC and got to be around many of the greats, like Marcus Allen, guys who took everything in stride, as well as a few guys who didn't deal with fame so well. I watched how they reacted to the limelight, and got to recognize certain patterns. I was able to see what worked and what didn't work, so when my time came I was ready.

> The first time I met Keyshawn, I was waiting in line at a burrito joint near the USC campus. A scuffle started between two groups of frat boys and one of the guys got knocked out. The police came and asked what happened, but the guy's buddies were scared and said they didn't know who'd hit him. Keyshawn was in line behind me and said, "Hey, that is your buddy! That is your friend and you are not going to help him? You know who just came in and did this and you are going to sit there and just tell the police that you don't know? That is your friend right there; you take care of him!" Then Key said, "I know who did it. Take me in your car and I'll go find him." And he went and found them and came back and got back in line and got his food.
>
> **Eric Espinoza, USC Assistant Strength Coach**

How do you handle fame? The key is to not forget who you are. Who you are and what you are is what got you here! Why should you change the way you are just because you became a success? Your energy, your attitude, and your commitment are reasons you became successful, so once you do become successful it is important for you to remain the same, to remain true to your values and your beliefs. The experiences of the past will help you solve present and future problems and help you see the best way for you to solve the challenges that lie ahead and to overcome the obstacles that life throws in your path. Material things around you may change, but your spiritual side should remain the same.

I use my past as a way to keep myself motivated, to remind myself during tough times exactly what I'm capable of. I say to myself, "My name is Keyshawn Johnson. I grew up in South Central L.A. It took a lot to get out of there and to reach where I am. They don't know what I went through to get here, but I do. I am not going to let anyone take away what I believe is mine. Not without giving it my all! If they are going to beat me, they are going to have to get up earlier than me and work harder than me, and that, my friend, they are not going to be able to do, because I will wake up before they wake up and work harder than them and in the end I will win!"

Your friends are one of the best links to your real self. Many of them were your friends before the fame, success, and wealth, and they are your friends now. You may not agree with the way some of them live or some of the things they do, but if they were by your side at your difficult times, they deserve to have you by their side when things are good for you. Just because success knocked at your door doesn't mean you can't or shouldn't relate to your old friends. Remember, the ones that were with you before will always be with you no matter what, so long as you are true to them, because they like you for what you are and not what you've become.

Success sometimes brings new challenges and new "friends." As a matter of fact, the more successful you become, the more difficult it is to sort out your real friends. Because with each step you climb on the ladder of success, a whole new group of people will want to become close to you and become a part of your success. There are a lot of people that want to be near success to absorb the positive energy that you give out. While some of these new people are going to become true friends, a good part of them just wants to take what you have to give, be it exposure, financial opportunities, or simply your energy. That is why the friends that you had before you became successful are so important, because you know they will be with you because of you and not because of your fame or success or money.

Your true friends are not only important because they are and have been a part of your history, they are also a source of grounding and good advice. Because they have been there with you before, they will be the ones to stop you and warn you, should you start losing touch with the real you. Many of your new "friends" are just going to be "yes" people, always ready to pump your ego up in an effort to get closer to you. But all they want is a part of you, and if some misfortune befalls you, they will be the first to abandon you and look for better pastures! You need those people like you need a pulled hamstring! Both will just slow you down.

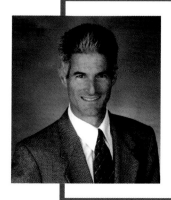

Keyshawn is a survivor and a self-made man. He did not have an easy life. He has earned everything he has achieved and has remained the same from his humble beginnings to today. Keyshawn has a lot of very strong characteristics. He is a very intelligent man, he is street smart, he can fit well with high-powered officers from the largest corporations in the world and with street kids and people from his old neighborhood.

Tim Tessalone, USC Sports Information Director

That being said, it does not mean that all new acquaintances are out to take advantage of you, or that all your old friends are going to remain the same and only have your best interests in mind. You need to exercise good judgment with *all* your acquaintances, especially once money and power enter the picture.

At times some bad experiences with newfound friends may make you want to stop letting new people into your life. That is a huge mistake! If someone wasn't smart enough to realize that being your friend is a precious thing and betrayed you, that's his problem! Don't let him change the way you are, otherwise you lose twice. Take these experiences as a lesson, become a better judge of people, but continue on being true to the essence of you, because happiness and success lie with being true to yourself and your values first!

I am very loyal to people. I probably shouldn't be as loyal as I am. If you do well with me you ought to do well in general. I've never had a problem reaching out and helping somebody. I don't understand people who aren't this way.

In life and in business, when you surround yourself with people you know, like, and trust, you greatly increase your chances for success. And who do you know better than your friends? When you create a great atmosphere, everyone is happy and puts forth their best effort. Remember, loyalty is a two-way street: your friends are loyal to you, and you give them back your loyalty. Together you are all stronger and tighter and are much more capable of overcoming obstacles than when alone!

Friendship is not something you learn in school. But if you haven't learned the meaning of friendship, you really haven't learned anything.
Muhammad Ali

10. Be Fit

You've got to be in top physical condition. Fatigue makes cowards of us all.
Vince Lombardi

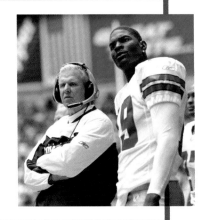

Keyshawn is a player that will attempt pretty much anything on the football field that you ask him to do. He's a tremendous blocker, probably one of the best two or three guys in football. And he will block anybody: defensive linemen, linebackers, defensive backs, anyone. You gain an appreciation for a player when he'll take on every task with the same amount of enthusiasm as he does pass receiving.

Bill Parcells

I've been around long enough to know that a successful wide receiver doesn't just catch the post patterns, he blocks and does all the other invisible things that help his team get into a position where they get a *shot* at a touchdown pass. I also know that I wouldn't be able to block or do the other little things well if I wasn't dead serious about my fitness program.

But being fit isn't just for professional athletes; a sound body is the basis for all your success in life, whether it's on the playing field or in the boardroom. Being strong, fit, and energized gives you the confidence to tackle anything. It even makes your mind work better! So far in this book I've given you the rules I live by. They help me make decisions and stay on the right track, no matter what life throws at me. Now it's time for me to tell you about the rest of the program: the workouts! Not only will they help you stay confident, but they'll ensure that other people give you the respect you deserve.

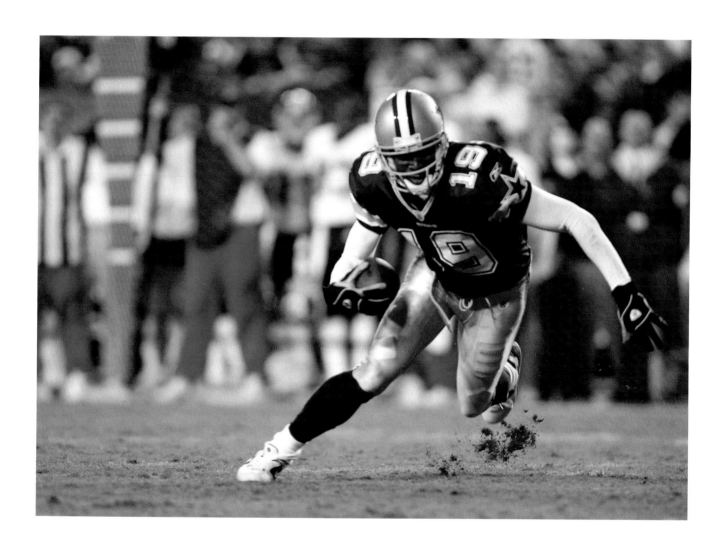

MEET THE AUTHORS

Keyshawn Johnson

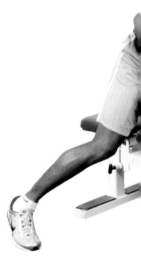

Keyshawn Johnson has achieved all the personal and team goals that a player can achieve in the National Football League. After being named the MVP of the Cotton Bowl as a junior for USC and the MVP of the Rose Bowl as a senior, in 1996 Keyshawn became the first wide receiver to be drafted #1 in the NFL since Irving Friar in 1984. A three-time All-Pro with the New York Jets and Tampa Bay Buccaneers, he won the Super Bowl with Tampa in 2002. Keyshawn combines his God-given talents with phenomenal physical conditioning and mental toughness. Playing the high-risk wide receiver position, Keyshawn only missed one game between 1997 and 2002 while averaging over 80 catches and 1000 yards receiving each season.

Keyshawn now plays for the Dallas Cowboys. In addition to his on-the-field heroics, he is a TV commentator, a successful businessman, and the owner of several restaurants in the Los Angeles, Tampa, and Dallas areas.

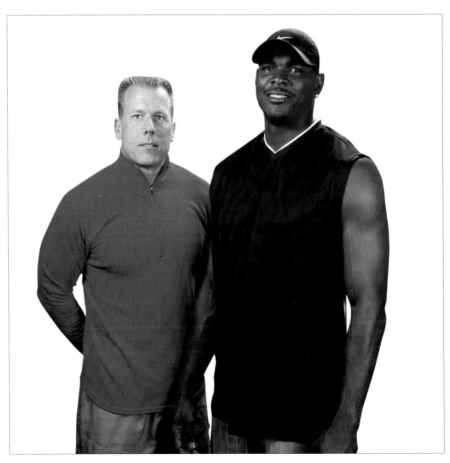

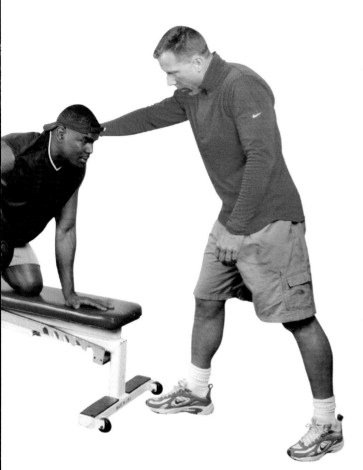

James Strom

James Strom began his strength coaching with the Los Angeles Rams in the 1980s, where he worked with Eric Dickerson, Jim Everett, and many other stars. From 1993 to 1998 he was head strength coach for the University of Southern California Trojans, where he was in charge of all nineteen varsity sports, both male and female. Some of the many athletes he worked with were basketball player Lisa Leslie, swimmer Janet Evans, and football players Keyshawn Johnson, Willie McGinest, Tony Boseli, and Jason Sehorn. In 1998 James became an exclusive private trainer. His clients have included football players Andre Rison and Keyshawn Johnson, actor Forrest Whitaker, and martial arts Ultimate Fighting Champion Royce Gracie. James teaches and lives in Los Angeles with his wife Jogie and daughter Sydney.

Kid Peligro

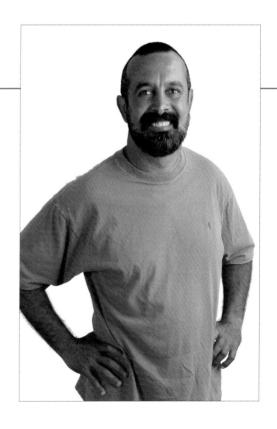

One of the leading martial arts writers in the world, Kid Peligro is responsible for regular columns in *Bodyguard* and *Gracie Magazine*, as well as one of the most widely read Internet MMA news page, *ADCC News*. A black belt in jiu-jitsu with two World Masters titles, Kid has been the author or coauthor of an unprecedented string of bestsellers in recent years, including *Superfit, The Gracie Way, Brazilian Jiu-Jitsu: Theory and Technique, Brazilian Jiu-Jitsu Self Defense Techniques, Brazilian Jiu-Jitsu Black Belt Techniques,* and *Brazilian Jiu-Jitsu Submission Grappling Techniques.* He makes his home in San Diego.

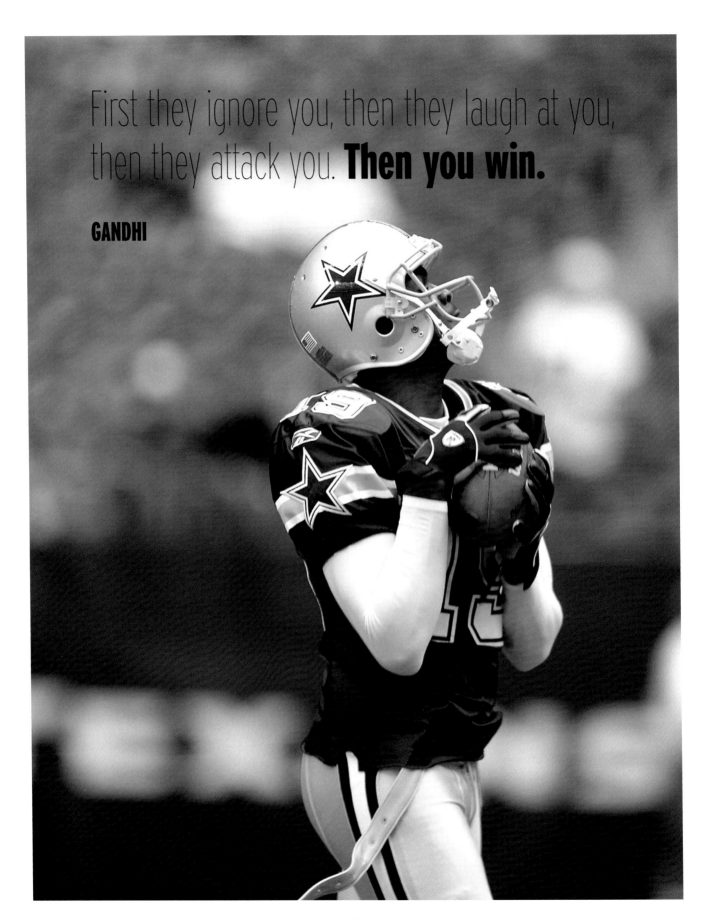

First they ignore you, then they laugh at you, then they attack you. **Then you win.**

GANDHI

PART ONE

WARMING UP AND STRETCHING

Being flexible enhances anyone's life, but for athletes it can mean the difference between victory and defeat. Their bodies are their instruments, and the ability to perform efficiently at their peak without injuries is paramount to a successful career. In general, a flexible person is not only less prone to injury, due to greater range of motion in muscles and joints, but also is able to deliver power more efficiently at a greater variety of angles and positions.

Additionally, with flexibility comes the ability to be comfortable and effective in situations where a less flexible person would struggle. There are three types of flexibility: static, functional, and ballistic. Static flexibility is the ability to get the most out of your range of motion in a slow, steady stretch. Functional flexibility involves stretching in one continuous motion while performing a task, such as twisting your torso in mid-air to catch the ball. Ballistic flexibility involves one's ability to reach the apex of the stretch in a ballistic—or explosive—situation, such as performing a throw or pitching a baseball. The stretches demonstrated in this book were developed specifically to meet the needs of everyone who must not only have excellent range of motion at rest but also be able to put that flexibility to work in functional and ballistic circumstances.

Just as flexibility varies from individual to individual, it also varies from joint to joint and side to side within an individual. A person may have very flexible hamstrings, for example, but be very stiff in the hips. No matter how flexible you are, significant improvement can be achieved with regular warm-ups and stretching exercises, such as the ones Keyshawn demonstrates here.

Warming Up

It is extremely important to warm up your joints and muscles prior to stretching or working out! Without proper warm-up, any attempt to stretch the "cold" joints and muscles may lead to injuries. Much as you let your car warm up before leaving your garage to make certain the oil has reached every bearing and valve in the engine, proper warm-up will "lubricate" your joints and muscle fibers with fresh blood and oxygen, assuring their best performance.

Pre-stretch warm-ups should consist of circling your hips, knees, and ankles while standing, followed by rotating each arm, circling your neck, and moving your head from side to side. Ideally, you should do a pre-stretch warm-up routine, then proceed to the Stretch Routine described below, followed by your workout and a second stretching session. This is especially important if you are preparing for a specific event such as a competition or a game. This program will not only give you power and explosion benefits but will also increase your ability to perform in a wide range of angles and motions. On those days when your time is really limited, you still need to squeeze the workout into your schedule if you want to progress. In this circumstance, you might consider dropping the stretch routines, but don't drop the warm-up! It is essential for keeping you from injury.

Stretching

The Stretch Routine presented here, when mastered, will render you more powerful, flexible, and less prone to injury. We recommend that you do the complete routine at least four times a week.

For all stretches, it is important to relax and breathe properly. The general rule of thumb is to exhale into your stretch. Do not bounce back and forth into any stretch except as noted, and do not push yourself beyond your limits! If you feel muscle or tendon pain when you are stretching, your body is telling you that you have reached your limit. Stop right there or even ease up a little, try to relax and breathe, and stay at that position for 30 seconds while you breathe and visualize your body part stretching. While you will reach "sticking" points in any stretch, your ability to breathe and to concentrate on relaxing the tight area will lead to steady progress.

One of the secrets of stretching is to progress slowly and listen to your body. If you haven't stretched in a while or are not sure how flexible you are, start slowly and progress slowly. You can accelerate your progress by stretching every day and by adjusting some of your daily movements to reflect the stretch routine. For example, if you have to pick something up from the ground, bend at the waist and stretch your hamstrings rather than bending at the knees and lowering your body. If you work a desk job, try placing one leg on the desk to stretch it while you talk on the phone, or try doing shoulder and neck stretches throughout the day. When you can do the beginner stretches easily, try the advanced. But always listen to your body before you commit to doing the advanced variations. Better to spend a little more time at the beginner level than risk injury by advancing too quickly. By following these principles you will improve your stretching naturally and seamlessly.

The Stretch Routine below is presented in the same order that Keyshawn performs it. He believes this to be the ideal sequence for himself and others, because you proceed from stretch to stretch and cover most of the muscles and joints involved in practicing sports and everyday life. We also present advanced options that require a spotter. Make sure you relax and breathe during all the stretches.

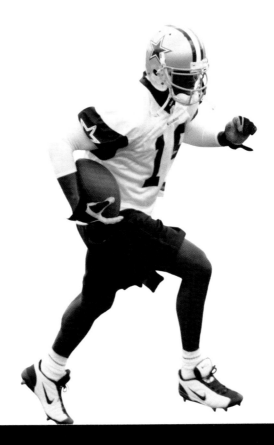

KEYSHAWN STRETCH ROUTINE

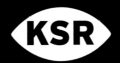

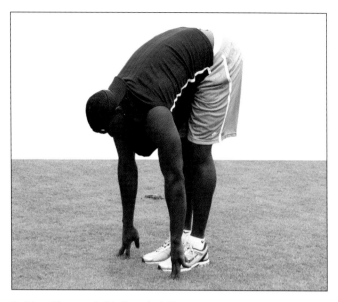

1. Standing upright, bend at the waist, and reach with your hands to touch your toes. If you cannot touch them, start by letting your arms dangle and let your body weight stretch your lower back. If you can touch easily, try putting the palms of your hands on the ground.

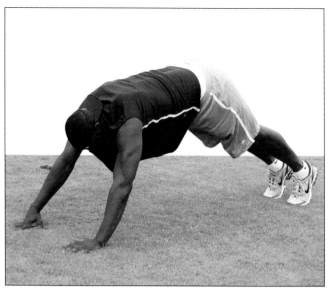

2. With your hands and feet on the ground, have your hips up, and press down as if you want to have your heels touch the ground to stretch your calves. You may switch the pressure from side to side as you stretch each calf.

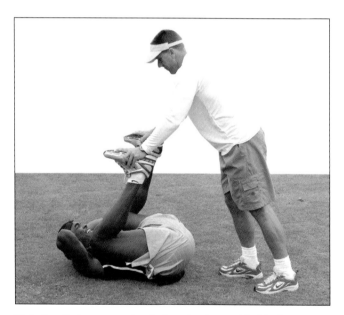

3. Lying flat on your back, hands clasped behind your head, bend your legs, and roll your knees toward your chest. **Advanced:** The spotter pushes down on your feet.

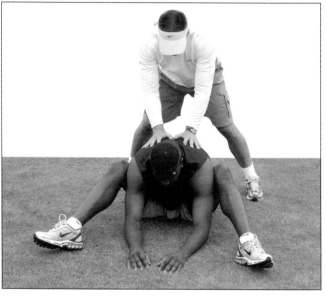

4. While seated on the ground, legs spread apart and knees bent, reach forward. Slowly move your hands forward (as if you were clawing the ground) as you continue the stretch. **Advanced:** The spotter applies pressure by pushing downward on the shoulder. Keep the pressure gentle and consistent. Stop at sticking points and push back against the pressure. Stretcher should then relax and stretch forward farther.

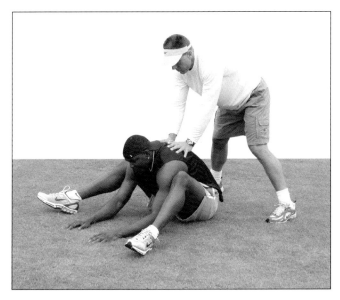

5. Maintain your stretching position by placing your elbows on the ground. **Advanced:** Continue until you can place your chest on the ground (very advanced).

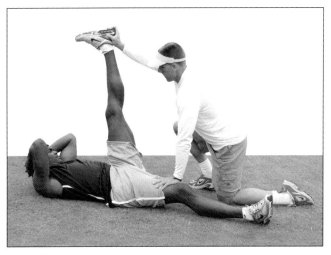

6. Lying with your back flat on the ground, keep both legs straight and bring one leg up, trying to touch your toes to the ground above your head. Hold the position when you feel slight muscle tension. Repeat with other leg. **Advanced:** Spotter presses down on the knee that is on the ground while pushing the other foot toward the head. If you do not have a spotter, you can use a towel. Wrap the towel around your upward pointing leg and pull on the ends of the towel to pull the leg toward your head.

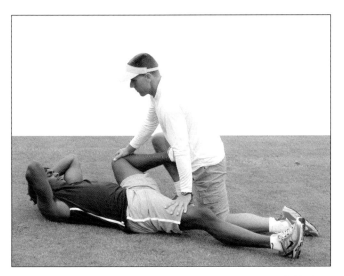

7. Lying flat on the ground, bend your leg and pull that knee toward your head. **Advanced:** Place your foot on the spotter's mid-section. The spotter should apply pressure by leaning forward. Make sure the spotter pushes down on the opposite knee to maximize the stretch.

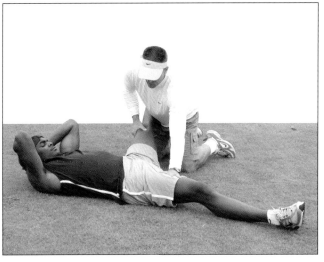

8. Lying with your back flat on the ground, keep your legs straight and open one leg out as you try to kick your own head. **Advanced:** Spotter holds the active leg 8-12 inches above the ground while applying pressure to the opposite leg. The spotter pushes the active leg upward. In the absence of a spotter, you can use a towel or a wall to assist the stretch.

KSR

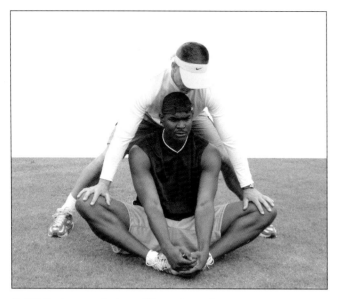

9. While in a seated position, place the soles of your feet together, clasp your hands around your toes, and lower your knees to the ground. **Advanced:** The spotter applies downward pressure by pushing down on the knees with his hands.

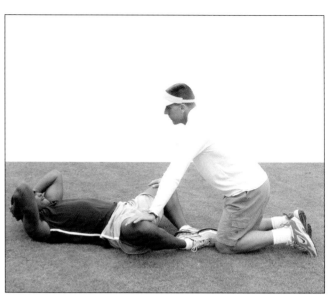

10. A variation of the previous stretch is to lie down flat on your back, hands clasped behind your head, chin tucked, and place the soles of your feet together.

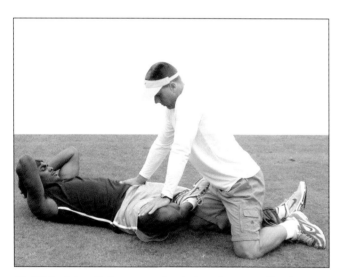

11. While lying flat on your back, bend your active leg upward and bring the knee to the ground. **Advanced:** The spotter places your foot on his thigh. While holding the opposite hip, the spotter pushes downward on the active leg.

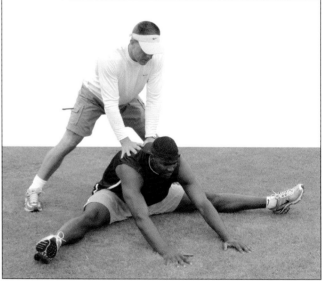

12. While seated on the ground, open your legs wide to a semi-comfortable position. Lean forward in front of you and reach with your hands and arms, bending your torso toward the ground. Claw forward with your hands on the ground to stretch farther. **Advanced:** The spotter applies additional pressure by pushing down on the shoulders. At sticking points, stop and push back against the pressure and then release for increased stretch. This is a great 3-in-1 stretch, as you engage the lower back, groin, and hamstring!

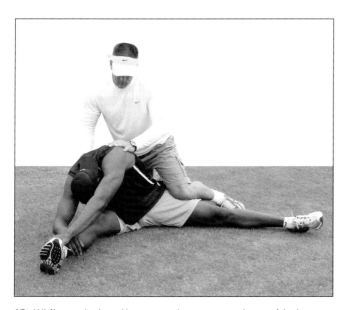

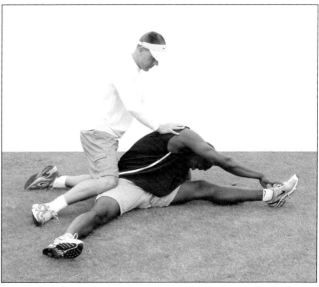

13. While seated on the ground, open your legs wide to a semi-comfortable position. Lean to one side as you reach to touch the toes with your hands. If you can't reach the toes, grab as far down as you can on the leg and slowly pull your torso down while walking your hands down the leg. If you reach your toes with your fingertips and want to further stretch, pull your toes back towards your head. **Advanced:** Spotter places his knee on the opposite leg to further force the stretch by keeping the hips on the ground.

14. Repeat step 13 on opposite side. It is important in all stretches to work both sides equally to maintain balance. Keep the nonactive leg flat and straight.

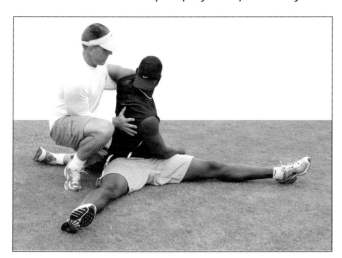

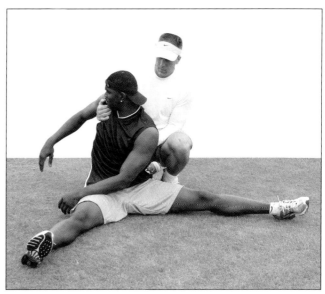

15. While seated on the ground, open your legs wide for balance and support. Twist your trunk to one side, reaching back around with the outside hand toward the opposite knee. Look toward the side you are turning to, letting your head aid in the twist. **Advanced:** The spotter reaches with his arm under the outside arm while applying pressure to the mid-back region with the other hand. Hold the position when you feel muscle tension. This is a great stretch for lower back rotation.

16. Repeat step 15 in the opposite direction. It is important to stay relaxed and keep your back straight.

KSR

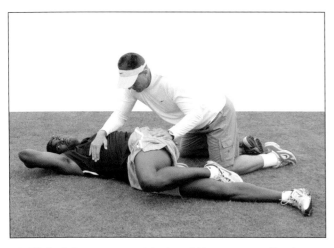

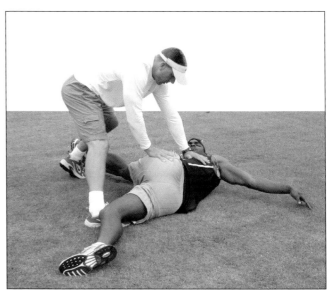

17. While lying on your side, bend the upper, active leg. Rest the foot behind the inactive down knee. Open your arm on the same side as the down knee and reach behind your head with your opposite hand. Keep your upper back flat on the ground and try to place your knee on the ground as your turn your hips. You may use the open hand to assist the stretch by pressing against the ground. **Advanced:** The spotter applies pressure by pushing gently on the hip and pulling on the chest, stretching the lower back region.

18. From the previous position, kick out the top leg, straightening it out for further stretch. Keep the down leg in a fixed position as much as possible. Make sure to relax and take deep breaths during the stretch. **Advanced:** The spotter moves the active leg upward while pushing on the hip and chest.

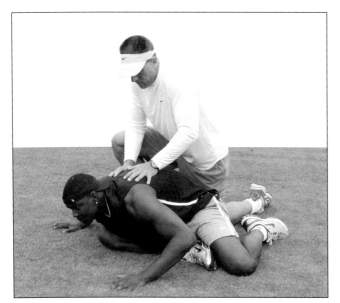

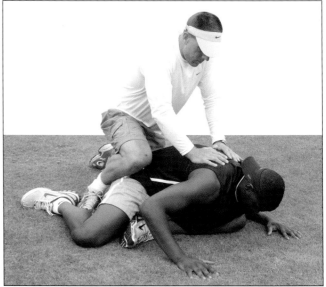

19. While in a semi-prone position, have your knees bent, with the active leg in front of you, and lower your chest to the ground. **Advanced:** The spotter applies pressure by pushing down on your back.

20. Repeat step 19, alternating the position of the legs. **Advanced:** This angle shows the spotter using his right leg to keep downward pressure on Keyshawn's right hip for further stretch.

PART TWO

THE EXERCISES

All sports exercises are complex moves that require most of the muscle groups in the body to perform in a coordinated fashion. Therefore, it is important to develop your muscles not only to be strong but also to be able to function in different planes of motion. The key is not simply muscle power but *functional* muscle power—the ability to deliver power in a rapidly changing environment. For example, a person who has trained strictly for power may be able to squat a tremendous amount of weight under perfect conditions in the gym. On the field, however, he wouldn't have the luxury of setting up for perfect form, and he may be unable to deliver the power when it is needed. An athlete with the proper sports training, on the other hand, should be able to adapt to the unpredictability of a game and be able to deliver power in less than ideal situations while still remaining in control of his actions and without injuring himself. A football player (wide receiver) such as Keyshawn may be running his route down the field and in an instant have to stop, cut and jump to adjust to the pass and to the defenders around him. That is *functional* muscle power, and it is what these exercises are designed to give you.

Breathing During the Exercises

Breathing is the most basic function of life. You can go a month without food or a couple of days without water, but more than a minute without oxygen and you are toast! Providing the muscles and brain with a rich supply of oxygen is essential in sports, where constant movement and stress tax the body, creating the need to breathe properly. If you learn to breathe correctly during the exercises, your ability will become apparent in your training and competing as well. The opposite is also true: improper breathing during workouts almost ensures ineffective breath in competition. Too often we see people simply inhale and try to retain the breath during an intense period of exercising, only to release the air all at once and be exhausted. In general, the correct way to breathe during exercising is as follows: *inhale* prior to the exertion, then *exhale* as you push the weight. Take a breath before you exert any energy and exhale as you exert it.

We are proud of the fact that our system emphasizes you, rather than specialized equipment. Anyone can take this book, make a few basic purchases, go in their garage, and do the workouts. With some dumbbells, a barbell, a jump rope, and some tubing, you can kick ass. Of course we do take advantage of machines as well. Machines are especially good for beginners and for extra strenuous exercises because of their stability.

Tips for Building *Our* Home Gym

Start small! You need some space dedicated to working out, the basic equipment listed below, this book, and motivation. That's it. To get yourself going as quickly and efficiently as possible, do these things:

- Consider your goals. Because our training is multidimensional, the program uses several simple types of equipment to make you fast, flexible, and powerful. To begin, you don't need a bunch of weights, tubes, or plyoballs, but you do need to be able to execute all the exercises. Get the basics and get started!

- Consider your space. Whether you plan to work out in your garage or your living room, you'll need room enough for stretching and ceilings high enough for jumping rope. Carpet will slow you down. Available space may influence your decision between fixed and solid weights.

- Consider your budget. Each item listed below can be had inexpensively, but—as with most things—you get what you pay for in exercise equipment. If your budget is limited, we recommend buying fewer pieces of good quality equipment and building as you can. A word to the wise: It pays to shop around!

- Look for hassle-free equipment. You want to be training, not fooling around with gear! Don't underestimate the value of customer service reps at specialty equipment stores. They are your best source of information in finding exactly the right equipment for you.

The Basics

If you prefer the convenience of working out at home, you'll need to purchase a few pieces of equipment. At minimum, you'll need:

> a flat bench
> a barbell
> a dumbbell set
> elastic tubing or a weight vest
> a jump rope
> a football
> medicine balls
> weight plates
> (if you use adjustable free weights)

When looking at flat benches, keep stability in mind. A basic 36-inch bench with 2-inch tubing will provide all the durability and security you can ask for. More expensive benches are adjustable, opening up your workout routines to include incline exercises.

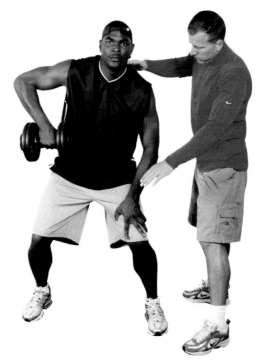

Free weights come in two varieties: fixed (also called solid) and adjustable (or pro-style). Fixed weights involve much less hassle as you switch from one exercise to another, but they are more expensive and can take up a great deal more room. If space is limited, we recommend going with a standard set of adjustable weights, which usually includes two dumbbell bars, a 5- or 6-foot barbell bar, weight clips, and around 110 lbs. of plates. At the very least, you'll want a few 2.5 lb. plates, a couple at 5 lbs., and a couple at 10 lbs. Broad, flat endcaps with permanent weight markings, although not necessary, will make your life a lot easier, and hex bolts fasten more securely than Allen bolts.

Elastic tubing is measured by the outside diameter and ranges from 1/8" to 1". You'll need to experiment a little to determine what works best for you, but we recommend that you start at least with the 1/4" tube and double it if you need extra power in the beginning. As you advance, you will need thicker tubes that you may have to double or triple, depending on your size and strength. As in selecting free weights, apply this rule of thumb: you need the load that will allow you to get through each exercise set but then make you struggle on the last repetition.

Medicine balls (also called plyoballs or body balls) come in leather, rubber, polyurethane, and vinyl. They are available in increments of 1 or 2 lbs., which gives you great versatility in choosing and increasing your load. Those that are filled with air or gel bounce when thrown against the ground or a wall, which can be very useful if you are training by yourself. Unlike free weights, medicine balls allow you to move in three dimensions, not only rotating, flexing, and extending, but also replicating explosive motions like throwing punches. These same benefits can create problems, so start slowly with a light medicine ball (between 4 and 8 lbs.) until you understand the power that they can develop. For grip strength, consider a 2 lb. ball.

Resources

Dumbbells, weights, and benches are best purchased at specialty exercise stores like Sportmart, Sports Authority, or Gart Brothers.

Elastics for the power series exercises can be found at scuba dive shops (they are used on spearguns) or online at places like **www.jumpusa.com** *or* **www.reefscuba.com.**

Harnesses (if you decide to purchase them) can be ordered online from **www.jumpusa.com.**

Medicine Balls can also be ordered from www.jumpusa.com or through **Century Martial Arts products (www.centuryma.com).**

Different Exercises and Their Purposes

To develop your functional muscle power, our system employs eight types of exercises: abdominal, cardiovascular, free weight, machine, isolateral, plyometric, Power Series and fieldwork. Each type of exercise is designed to work a particular part of the body or to prepare you for a particular aspect of sports competition.

As we explain in greater detail later, our system encourages you to experiment by altering the workouts. This will prevent them from becoming stale and ensure that you stay focused and challenged. To help you modify the workouts, each exercise in the workout routines is marked with an icon that refers to the categories of exercises below. Using the icons, you can easily replace exercises from one category with others from the same category, giving you great flexibility without any guesswork!

Let's take a few minutes to consider each category of exercise.

AB Abdominal Exercises

In highly physical performance sports such as football, gymnastics, explosiveness, speed, and power come ultimately from your center—your abdominals. Whether positioning your body to execute a move, striking with your arms or legs, or blocking, parrying, or absorbing a blow, your abdominal strength is critical to your effectiveness. The core (the center area of your body comprising the abdomen and your lower back) connects your upper body to your lower body and is responsible for transferring power and explosiveness from one area to the next. Obviously the more conditioned and fit your core is, the better you will perform not only in sports but in day-to-day physical activities. A rock-hard midsection not only gives you the advantage of stability as you move, but it also protects the most vulnerable part of your body. Special attention given to conditioning your abs will pay off in greater performance and increased protection.

Our workouts challenge you to work your abs every day you exercise. But don't think we expect you just to grit your teeth through an endless number of crunches. We've provided a range of exercises that will keep you interested, keep you challenged, and make your midsection the powerful, elastic core serious athletes need.

CC Cardiovascular Conditioning

Cardiovascular exercises increase your ability to pump blood and process oxygen. Typically, they involve low-impact, large muscle movement over a sustained period of time, which raises your heart rate to 50 percent or more of its maximum level. Examples of cardiovascular exercises include running, walking, stair climbing, and swimming. Benefits from cardiovascular exercise include lowering blood pressure, increasing HDL (good) cholesterol, decreasing LDL (bad) cholesterol, along with increased heart and lung function and efficiency and decreased anxiety, tension, and depression. The National Institute on Aging (NIA) states, "Endurance activities help prevent or delay many diseases that seem to come with age. In some cases, endurance activity can also improve chronic diseases or their symptoms." Cardiovascular capacity is not only a major component of feeling good and being healthy, it is also vital for all competitors. If you tire during a competition or a game, you are doomed. Your ability to perform is directly related to your cardiovascular conditioning.

FW Free-Weight Exercises

Machines are very stable and are good for the development of specific muscles, but they don't imitate real life very well. We only use machines for specific exercises for which machines are best suited; otherwise we prefer free weights. When you use a barbell, you introduce an element of instability that engages different muscles. When you go one step further and introduce dumbbells in each hand, you increase the instability factor and make it even more difficult to balance and control the weights. This accomplishes two things:

First, you develop your "stabilizers" and "neutralizers." These are two groups of muscles whose objective is to balance and control. Many athletes develop very strong muscles, but unless they have equally capable neutralizers and stabilizers, they will develop joint problems because their joints cannot withstand their newly acquired power. This risk is amplified by the rigors of sports like football, basketball, and martial arts, which demand maximum ranges of both power and motion in the joints.

Second, using free weights develops your motor coordination and challenges your brain to stay in the exercise. When you exercise with a machine, the axis and steel of the machine allow the weight to move only in a prescribed manner; therefore, you can exercise almost without engaging your brain. With the free weights, you must always maintain focus on your actions or you may lose control of the weight. This causes you to tire more quickly, but challenging your body with these additional variables stimulates and trains your muscles, as well as your neuromuscular system, to perform better and longer.

Another problem with training on machines is that you may not find the equipment you are used to or need for your specific program when you are traveling in another city or country. Every gym, however, has dumbbells and barbells, and it's easy enough to pack a rope and some elastic wherever you go. So no matter where you go you can execute the majority of your workout and all you need are the basic things found in even the most humble gym.

ME Machine Exercises

Machines exercises are very effective as a complement to free weights and develop some muscles well. As we stated above, machines, because of their stability and safety, are especially good for high loads and for beginners, seniors, and recuperating athletes. Because of their controlled motion and ability to isolate certain muscle groups, they allow you to use heavier loads and to track progress much more easily than free weights.

(ISO) Isolateral Exercises

Isolaterals are exercises designed to balance your muscular structure. Typically, they involve working one limb or one side of the body at a time while performing conventional exercises like the bench press, military press, or upright row. In the bench press with dumbbells, for example, you would hold one weight steady in one hand while performing the exercise with weight in the other.

Our system involves doing a number of isolateral repetitions to one side and then changing sides and repeating the routine on the other side—not necessarily for the same number of repetitions. This balances your muscle power. Since most people have a dominant side, isolateral exercises can be adjusted to create balance. For instance, if your right side is dominant, you can do 10 reps on the right and 15 on the left. This will give you greater ability to react and execute moves to both sides. Isolaterals close up such weaknesses.

(PL) Plyometric Exercises

Our system uses quite a few exercises that involve plyometrics—quick bursts that repeatedly stretch and contract your muscles. Plyometric exercises are perfect for everyone because they connect explosive movement with power and strength, enhancing your ability to perform under realistic conditions. By training your body to move with quickness and agility, you will gain both. Being able to deliver power at the precise instant it's needed in an active environment is exactly what athletes require. Take, for instance, a wrestler attempting to execute a takedown. First, he coils his body in anticipation of the attack, then he lunges forward at his opponent until he secures the proper grip. At that instant, he must be able to switch once again to using power and speed to take the opponent down. Or watch Keyshawn sprinting down the field to catch the ball. In a split second, he may need to transform the energy of the spring into a leap while extending his arm to catch the football. Perhaps you are not a football player. You may still need to jump and catch your child before he hits the ground if he has tripped or she has jumped on you without warning!

If you concentrate simply in specific aerobic conditioning and weight training exercises, you are only preparing yourself to endure and to apply power in a static environment, which is the furthest thing from the realities of sports. In sports and sometimes in real life, you are required not only to have stamina and strength, but also to be able to react to the opportunities or demands that arise during a competition against a living, thinking opponent. Plyometrics are the key to developing such "reactionary instincts" in your muscles.

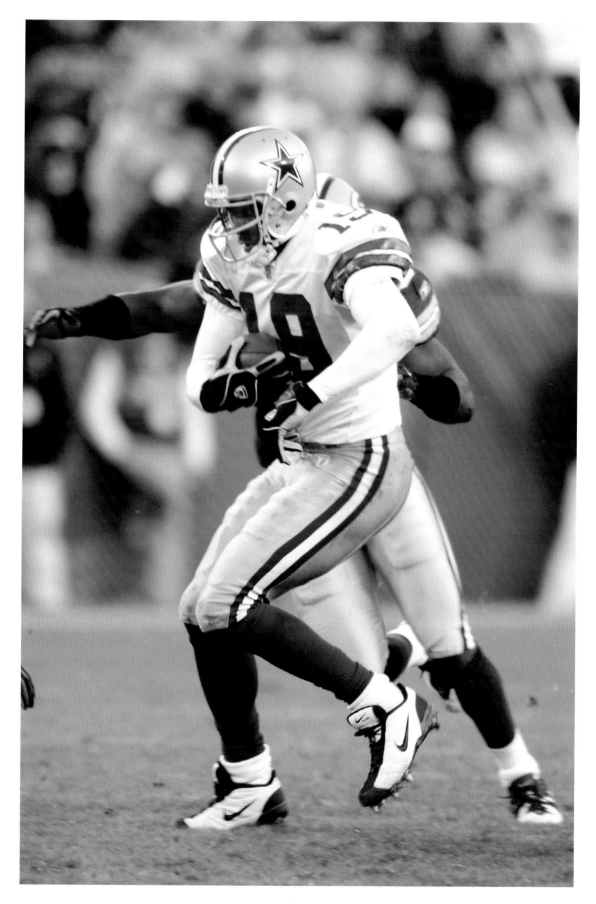

In this book you will be shown a variety of plyometric exercises such as the box jumps (59), the lateral jumps (61), and some of the medicine ball exercises. Typically in plyometrics, one attempts to perform the greatest number of repetitions in a set period of time without losing form. For that reason these exercises not only challenge your explosion and coordination, but they also increase your stamina and endurance.

A word of caution: plyometrics are high-impact exercises and as such they may aggravate conditions such as tendonitis, arthritis, and bursitis. Make sure you maintain proper form while doing plyometrics. If you begin to tire and lose form, stop immediately. If you practice after your form is lost, you will only be training yourself to execute improper techniques. Losing form is your signal to take a break.

Power Series Exercises

Our power series exercises are power-building exercises that take plyometrics to the next level. Like plyometrics, the power series typically (with some exceptions like the static wall sit) involve a quick, explosive movement, and the key to the exercises is to begin with little or no pressure and concentrate on form, explosion, and speed. What you want is to do the greatest number of repetitions in a certain amount of time without compromising technique. If you start to lose form, stop.

What distinguishes the power series exercises is their unique attention to combining cardiovascular fitness and muscular strength while replicating real-life movements vital for athletes—lateral motions and explosive motions like cutting, hitting, jumping, and sprinting. To achieve this combination, many of the exercises involve the use of a harness and elastic cords (or a weight vest) to create progressive resistance. As you master each exercise and reach reasonable speed, increase your resistance or have your spotter add pressure. You'll increase your endurance and your strength at the same time.

Fieldwork Exercises

Fieldwork exercises were specially developed by James Strom to increase agility, coordination, stamina, cardiovascular capacity, explosion, and reaction time. The fieldwork exercises are both challenging and fun while putting you through a rigorous workout. By using movement in conjunction with specific tasks, these exercises will take you through a variety of motion that will use just about every muscle and tendon in your body.

Fieldwork exercises are a combination of plyometrics, power series, and simple agility drills.

Common Training Mistakes

The American Council of Exercise points out 5 mistakes that people make while exercising. Pay attention and avoid them.

1. **Using bad form** – As we pointed out above, you should not continue or even start exercising without proper form. If you are in the middle of a set and your form begins to suffer because you are tired, you should stop immediately. Repeating exercises without proper form teaches you to do them wrong and trains your muscles to replicate the motion incorrectly, leading to injuries.

2. **Pursuing an unbalanced strength-training program** – Our system is designed to stimulate and increase your capacity in all the muscle groups. Many people err by addressing only a certain area of their bodies, like they'd like to have stronger legs, so they concentrate on squats. Their focused efforts, however, may lead to an unbalanced body, postural problems, and pain from improper muscle balance. In another example, a person may be focused on developing a perfect set of abs and concentrate on those while ignoring the lower back muscles. The abs then grow stronger and pull the torso forward without proper compensation from the lower back muscles, creating a postural misalignment and back problems. The same type of problem can occur if you overdeveloped your hamstrings without balancing the strength of your quadriceps. The hamstrings will pull the back of your hips without compensation from the quadriceps and again you will have misalignment and back problems.

3. **Progressing unwisely** – Many people fail to achieve progress because they do not follow a properly designed exercise routine. By following our exercise program and allowing proper rest, you will achieve the results you want

4. **Failing to provide enough variety** – Unlike most exercise programs, we do not focus on one or two muscle groups each day. Rather, we engage many—if not all—muscle groups at each workout because in regular life and in sports you are continually required to use all the muscles. Additionally, our system is designed with great flexibility and variation to stimulate you and your body to achieve progress in the face of constant challenge.

5. **Failing to cool down properly after your workout** – It is very common for people to feel so good that they have finished their workout that the last thing they want to do is to cool down. Cooling down, however, is very important. You should take the time to stretch the muscles that you've used. This will increase your flexibility and will also get you energized for your next workout.

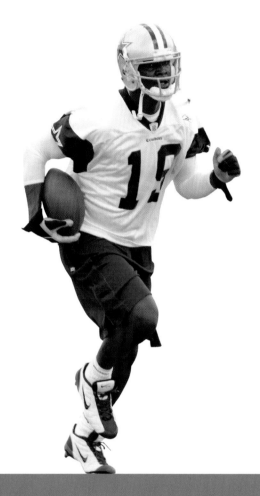

ABDOMINALS

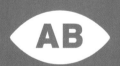

1. High Crunches

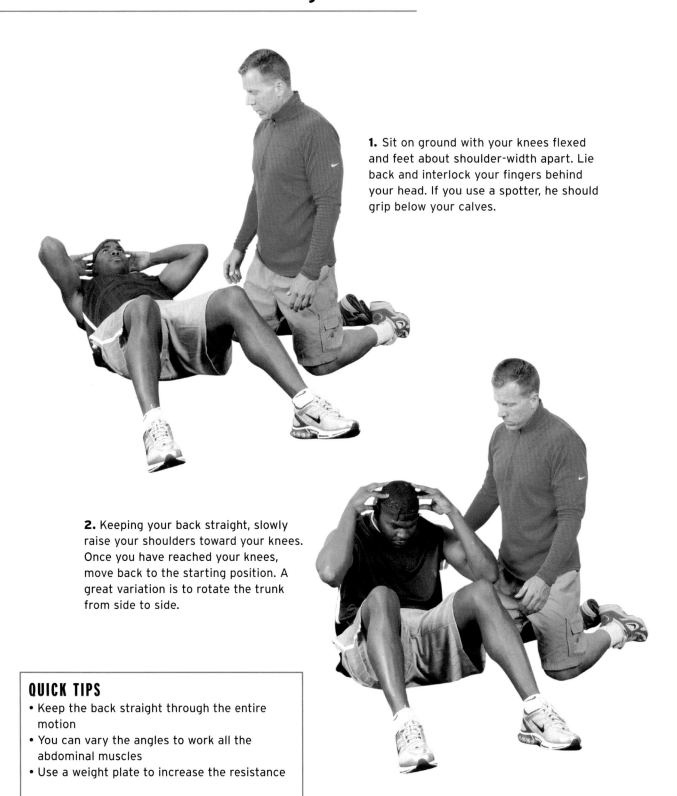

1. Sit on ground with your knees flexed and feet about shoulder-width apart. Lie back and interlock your fingers behind your head. If you use a spotter, he should grip below your calves.

2. Keeping your back straight, slowly raise your shoulders toward your knees. Once you have reached your knees, move back to the starting position. A great variation is to rotate the trunk from side to side.

QUICK TIPS
- Keep the back straight through the entire motion
- You can vary the angles to work all the abdominal muscles
- Use a weight plate to increase the resistance

2. Good Mornings

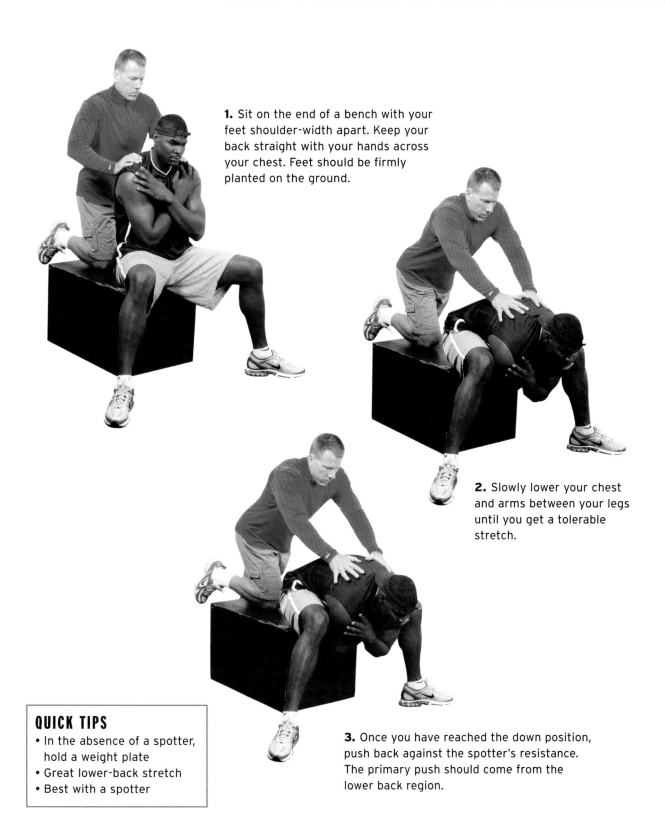

1. Sit on the end of a bench with your feet shoulder-width apart. Keep your back straight with your hands across your chest. Feet should be firmly planted on the ground.

2. Slowly lower your chest and arms between your legs until you get a tolerable stretch.

3. Once you have reached the down position, push back against the spotter's resistance. The primary push should come from the lower back region.

QUICK TIPS
- In the absence of a spotter, hold a weight plate
- Great lower-back stretch
- Best with a spotter

AB

3. Good Mornings with Twist

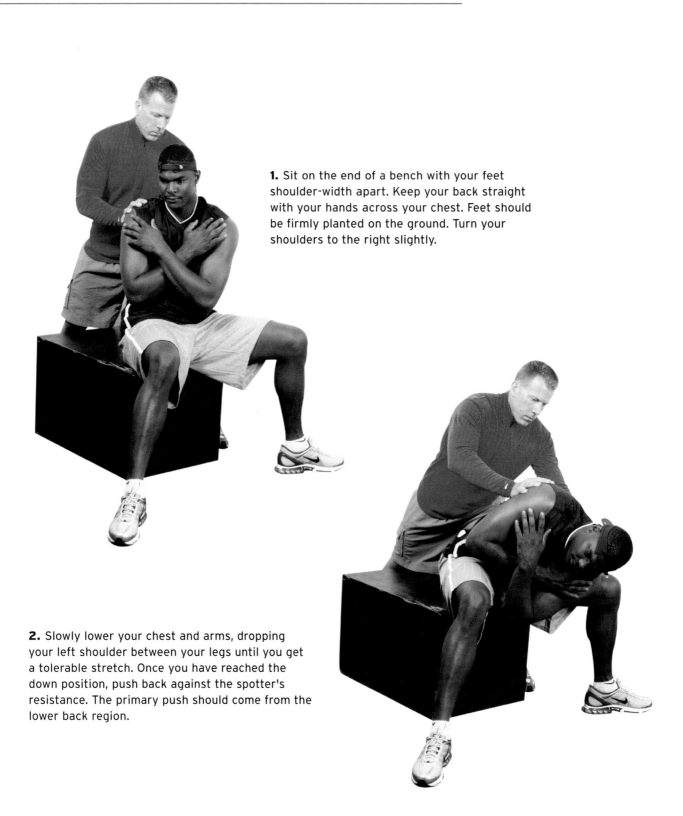

1. Sit on the end of a bench with your feet shoulder-width apart. Keep your back straight with your hands across your chest. Feet should be firmly planted on the ground. Turn your shoulders to the right slightly.

2. Slowly lower your chest and arms, dropping your left shoulder between your legs until you get a tolerable stretch. Once you have reached the down position, push back against the spotter's resistance. The primary push should come from the lower back region.

4. Roll-Ups

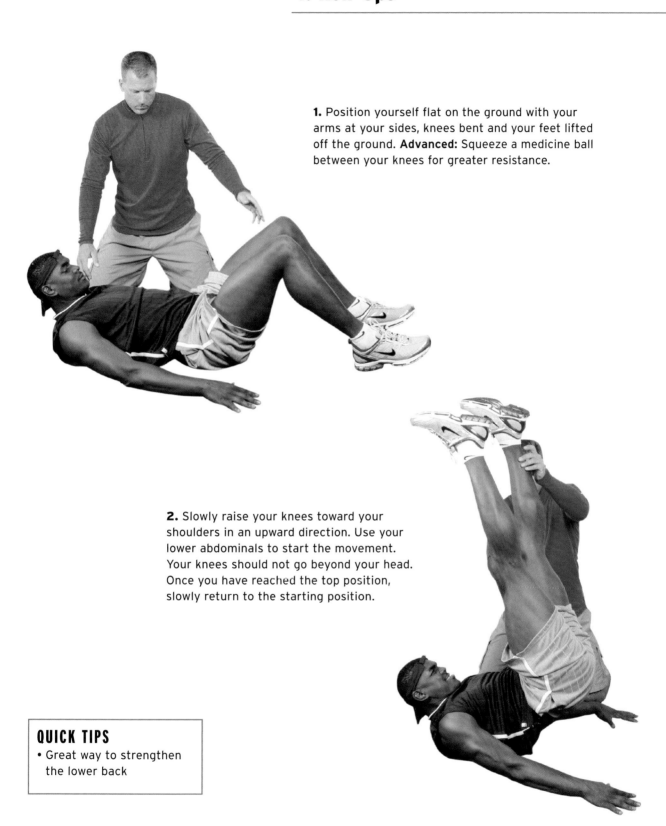

1. Position yourself flat on the ground with your arms at your sides, knees bent and your feet lifted off the ground. **Advanced:** Squeeze a medicine ball between your knees for greater resistance.

2. Slowly raise your knees toward your shoulders in an upward direction. Use your lower abdominals to start the movement. Your knees should not go beyond your head. Once you have reached the top position, slowly return to the starting position.

QUICK TIPS
• Great way to strengthen the lower back

AB

5. V-Ups

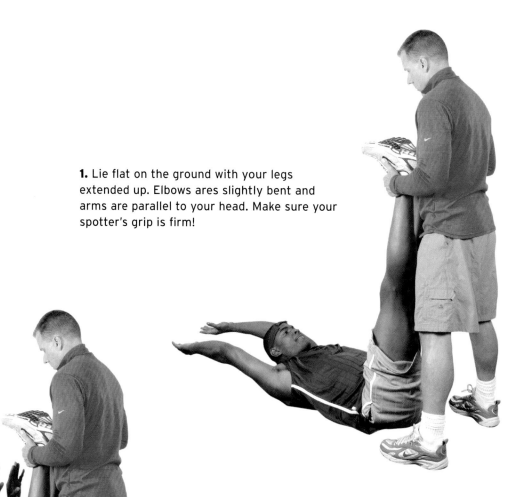

1. Lie flat on the ground with your legs extended up. Elbows ares slightly bent and arms are parallel to your head. Make sure your spotter's grip is firm!

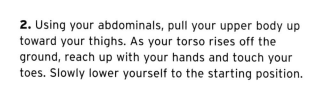

2. Using your abdominals, pull your upper body up toward your thighs. As your torso rises off the ground, reach up with your hands and touch your toes. Slowly lower yourself to the starting position.

QUICK TIPS
• Must have a spotter
• Good for lower back as well as abs
• Intermediate/Advanced

6. Bent Leg Crunch with Twist

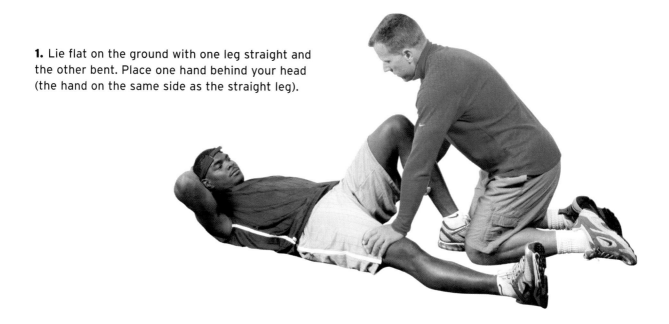

1. Lie flat on the ground with one leg straight and the other bent. Place one hand behind your head (the hand on the same side as the straight leg).

2. Rise up in a semi-seated position. As you move upward, bring your bent elbow across your body, touching the knee of your bent leg. Repeat on other side.

AB

7. Decline Bench Crunch with Medicine Ball

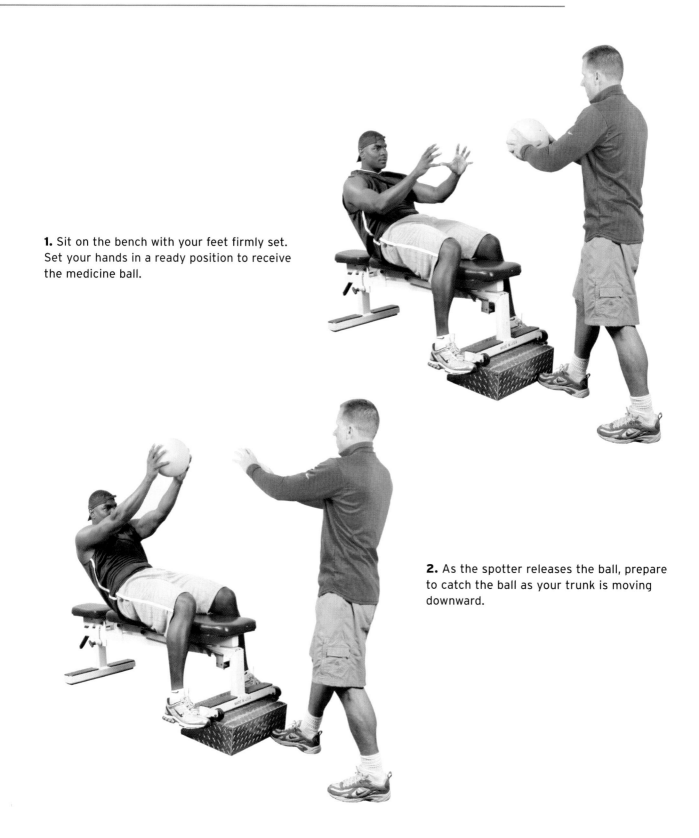

1. Sit on the bench with your feet firmly set. Set your hands in a ready position to receive the medicine ball.

2. As the spotter releases the ball, prepare to catch the ball as your trunk is moving downward.

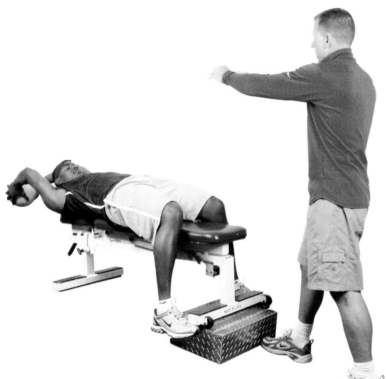

3. Let the momentum of the ball push your trunk downward and carry your arms over your head. Once your back is straight, raise your arms and trunk upward, tossing the ball back to your partner.

4. Toss the ball to the spotter and get set to repeat.

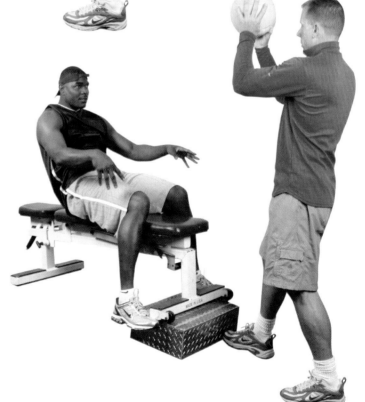

QUICK TIPS
• Always descend in a controlled manner

AB

8. Decline Bench Medicine Ball Hold and Twist

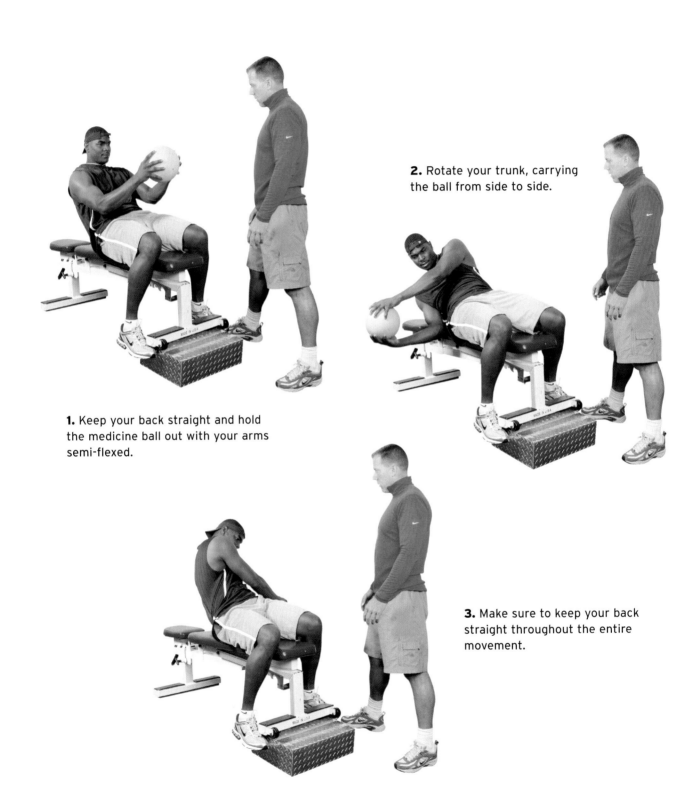

2. Rotate your trunk, carrying the ball from side to side.

1. Keep your back straight and hold the medicine ball out with your arms semi-flexed.

3. Make sure to keep your back straight throughout the entire movement.

9. Decline Bench Medicine Ball Toss with Twist

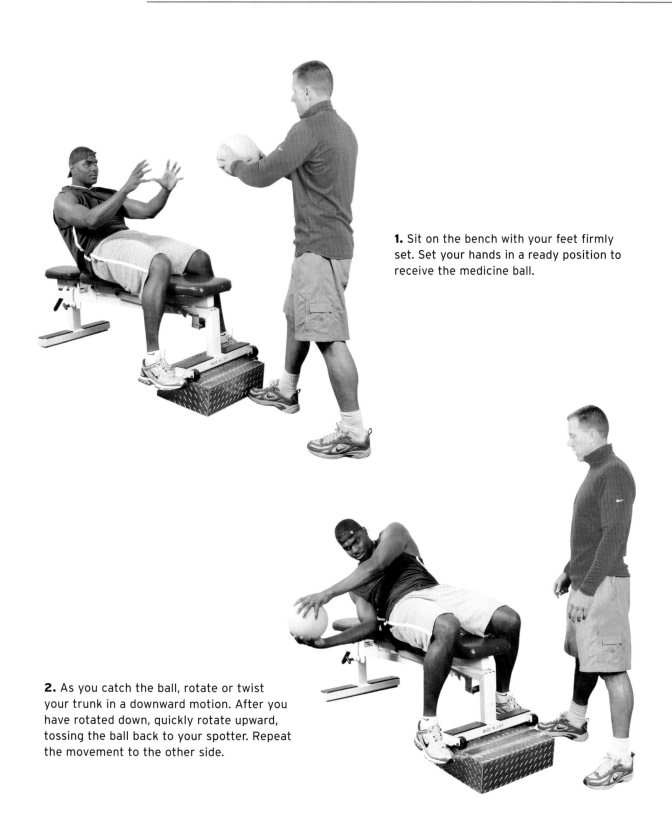

1. Sit on the bench with your feet firmly set. Set your hands in a ready position to receive the medicine ball.

2. As you catch the ball, rotate or twist your trunk in a downward motion. After you have rotated down, quickly rotate upward, tossing the ball back to your spotter. Repeat the movement to the other side.

AB

10. Medicine Ball Plyometric Oblique Toss

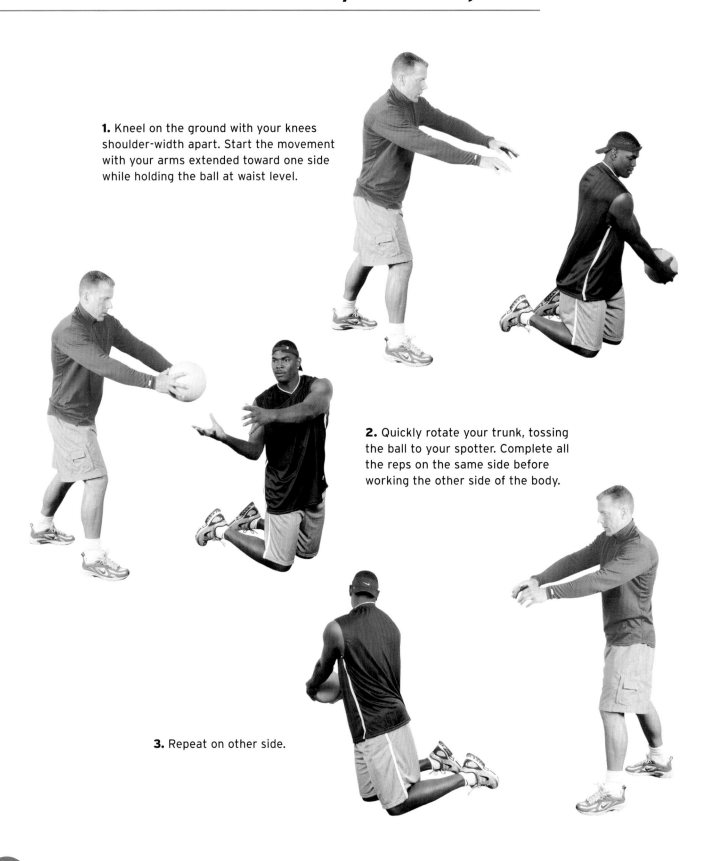

1. Kneel on the ground with your knees shoulder-width apart. Start the movement with your arms extended toward one side while holding the ball at waist level.

2. Quickly rotate your trunk, tossing the ball to your spotter. Complete all the reps on the same side before working the other side of the body.

3. Repeat on other side.

11. Leg Throws

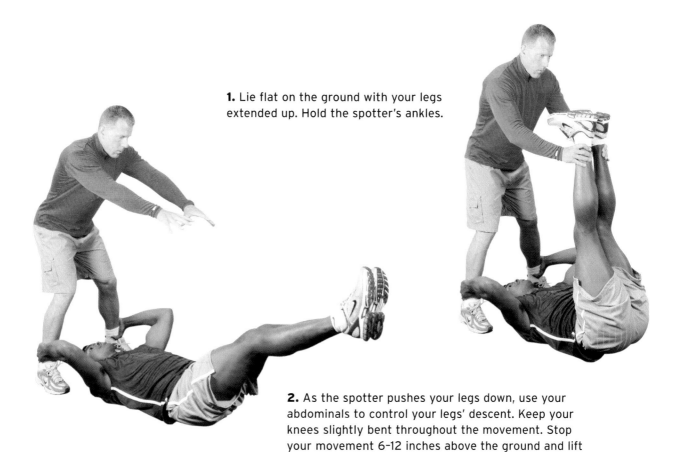

1. Lie flat on the ground with your legs extended up. Hold the spotter's ankles.

2. As the spotter pushes your legs down, use your abdominals to control your legs' descent. Keep your knees slightly bent throughout the movement. Stop your movement 6–12 inches above the ground and lift your legs back to the starting point.

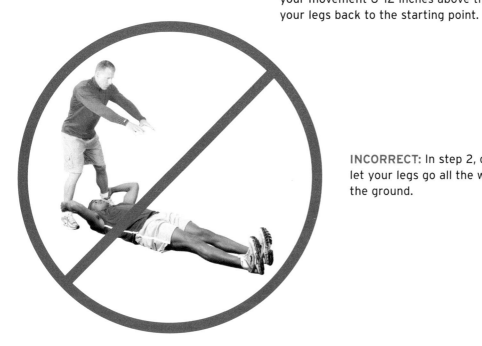

INCORRECT: In step 2, do not let your legs go all the way to the ground.

AB

12. Knee-Ups

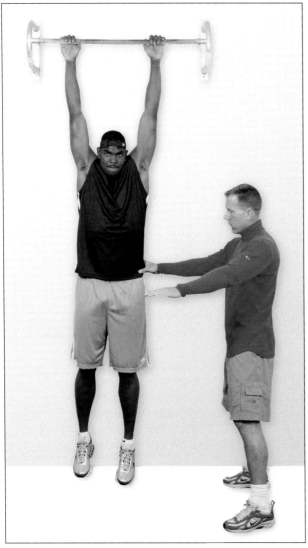

1. Grab a pull-up bar with your hands.

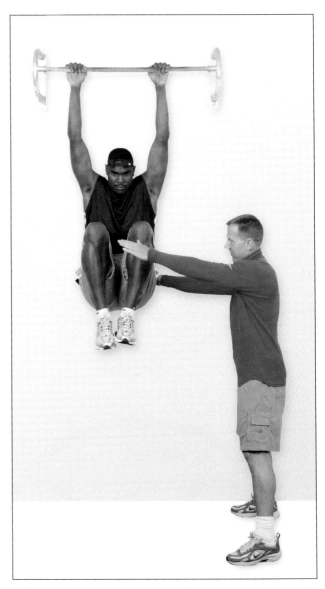

2. Keeping your arms extended, raise your knees until they touch your chest. Lower and start over.

QUICK TIPS
- Great for abs, grip strength, and endurance
- You can use a towel to add grip strength
- For added difficulty, trap a medicine ball between the legs and raise knees until it touches chest

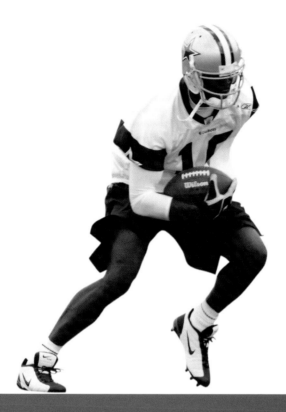

CARDIOVASCULAR CONDITIONING

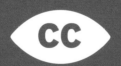

The exercises on this page are familiar enough that they need no demonstration. Use your own judgment and experience in setting them up to best serve your needs.

13. Jump Rope

Beginner: Start with both feet together and jump rope in place.
Intermediate: Every third jump, try to jump extra high through the rope.
Advanced: Get in a squat stance and jump rope.

14. Run in Place

Run in place while your spotter controls the pressure with a harness.

15a. Soft Sand or Grass Run

Run in soft sand for length of time specified by workout. If running on sand is not an option, run in grass for upper limit of time specified. If sand or grass is not an option, see 15b.

15b. Steady Run or Jog

Run or jog for length of time specified by workout.

16. Sprints

Sprint distance specified at 70-80% intensity unless otherwise noted. Walk or jog back to starting place.

17. Run and Hold

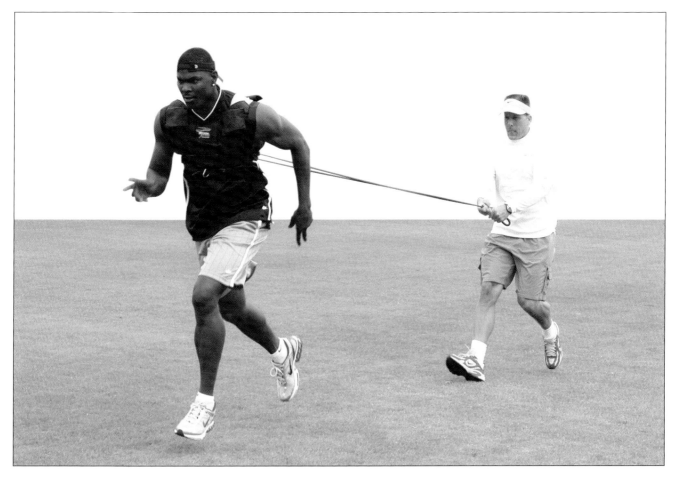

1. Similar to running in place but spotter lets you run a certain distance and holds you in place for a set number of seconds.

QUICK TIPS
- Great for balance and explosive strength
- Great for endurance and agility
- Use weight vest instead of bungee if no spotter is available
- Use different distances and thicknesses of bungee cord to vary the resistance
- Concentrate on form and speed
- If form suffers, stop the exercise and rest

CC

18. Resistance Running

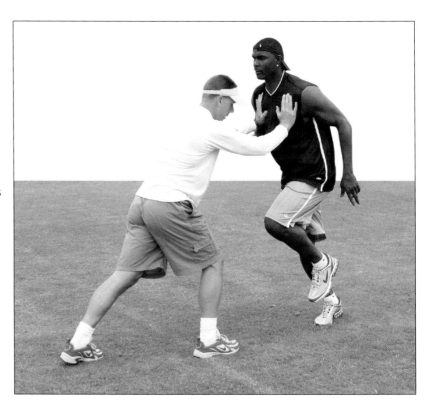

1. Stand in a split stance in front of your spotter. The spotter should place his hands on your chest.

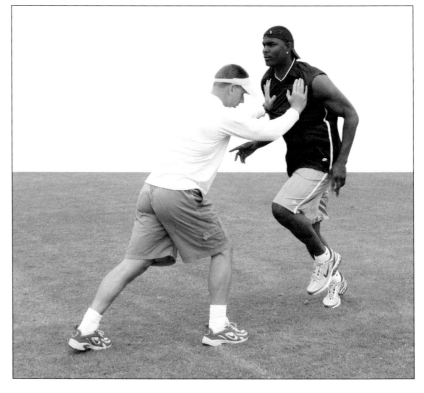

2. Start running forward while the spotter provides resistance.

19. Explosive Running

1. This drill requires some type of harness and cord to add resistance. Position your body and feet so you can quickly accelerate.

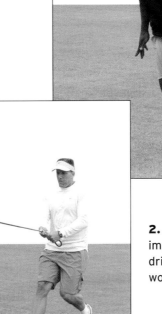

2. Accelerate in a straight line. It is important to use your arms and legs to drive yourself forward to generate working speed.

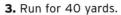

3. Run for 40 yards.

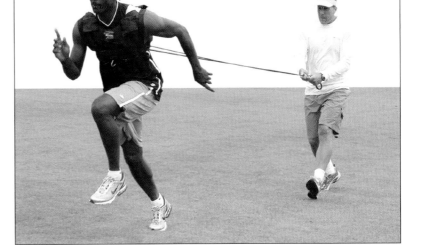

CC

20. Treadmill Workouts/Protocols

Keyshawn is a firm believer in treadmills. He has been running on them since his USC days and uses them regularly as part of his training regimen. Treadmills offer great advantages over street running for most people, including:

- Excellent opportunity to develop proper running form
- Less impact and less stress on the joints
- Power to control the degree of incline
- Capacity to monitor running speed and vary it (up to 12 mph) to meet individual needs
- Opportunity to create individualized workouts
- Freedom from uncomfortable weather like rain or snow

Protocol A

Time	Speed (mph)	Incline
3 minutes	6	0%
1-minute rest		
2 minutes	7	0%
45-second rest		
1 minute	8	0%
30-second rest		
45 seconds	9	0%
30-second rest		
30 seconds	10	0%

Repeat last step 6 times, 30 seconds @ 10 mph, 0% incline, with 30-second rests between reps.

Protocol B

Time	Speed (mph)	Incline
2 minutes	6	0%
45-second rest		
2 minutes	7	0%
45-second rest		
1 minute	8	0%
30-second rest		
45 seconds	10	0%
20-second rest		
20 seconds	12	0%

Repeat last step 6 times, 20 seconds @ 12 mph, 0% incline, with 20-second rests between reps.

Protocol C

Time	Speed (mph)	Incline
2 minutes	6	2%
30-second rest		
1 minute	7	2%
30-second rest		
1 minute	8	4%
30-second rest		
30 seconds	9	4%
30-second rest		
30 seconds	10	6%
30-second rest		
20 seconds	12	6%

Repeat last step 8 times, 20 seconds @ 12 mph, 6% incline, with 20-second rests between reps.

Protocol D

Time	Speed (mph)	Incline
1 minute	6	1%
30-second rest		
1 minute	7	2%
30-second rest		
30 seconds	7.5	3%
30-second rest		
30 seconds	8	4%
30-second rest		
30 seconds	8.5	5%
30-second rest		
30 seconds	9	6%
30-second rest		
30 seconds	9.5	7%
30-second rest		
30 seconds	10	10%

Repeat last step 6–8 times, 30 seconds @ 10 mph, 10% incline, with 30-second rests between reps.

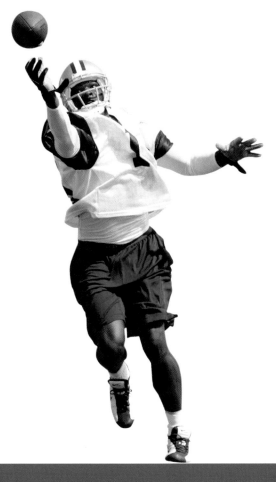

FREE WEIGHTS

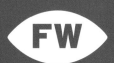

21. Bench Press-Barbell

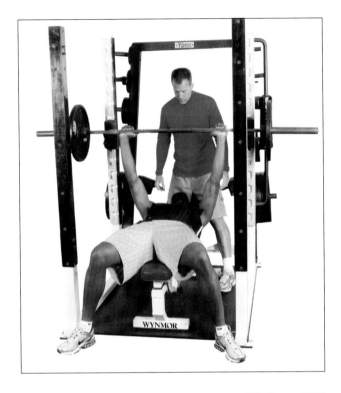

1. Your grip should be equal, your elbows straight, and your shoulders and buttocks should touch the bench. Your feet are flat on the floor.

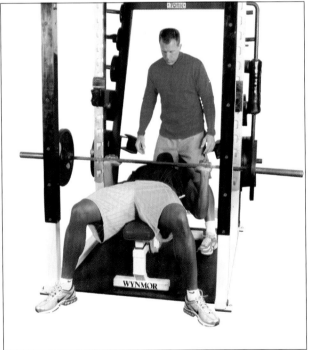

2. The descent of the bar is controlled. The bar should gently touch your sternum as you prepare to press the barbell back to the starting position. Keeping your feet and buttocks firmly planted, push the barbell back to the starting position.

QUICK TIPS
• Slightly arch your lower back
• Always keep your buttocks on the bench
• Use a spotter

22. Bench Press–Dumbbell

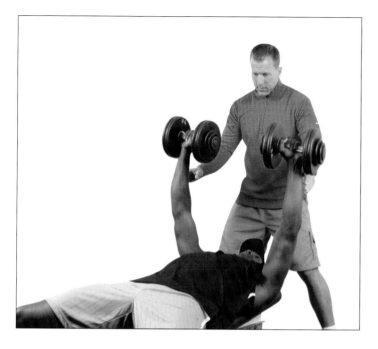

1. Hold a dumbbell in each hand, palms facing forward. Make sure your feet are firmly planted on the ground and keep a solid base. Your back should be slightly arched, with your buttocks on the bench.

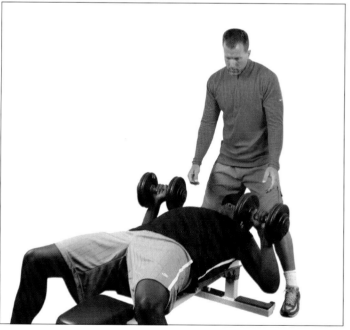

2. Lower the dumbbells in an equal, controlled motion until they touch the outer chest area. At this point, press the dumbbells back to the starting position.

QUICK TIPS
• Rest the dumbbells on your thighs before starting
• Always start at the top with the arms extended

FW

23. Front Raise-Dumbbell

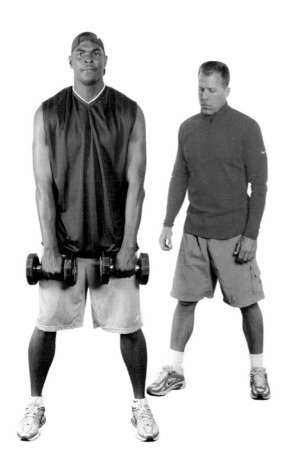

1. Stand erect with feet shoulder-width apart, holding a dumbbell in each hand.

2. Raise the dumbbell to eye level. Hold for 1-2 seconds at the top end, then slowly return to the starting position.

QUICK TIPS
• Great exercise to strengthen the anterior deltoid

24. High Pull-Dumbbell

1. Your stance should be wider than shoulder width and your feet flat on the ground. Your knees are bent and your thighs should be parallel to the ground. Use a closed grip and position the dumbbell between your legs, slightly off the ground.

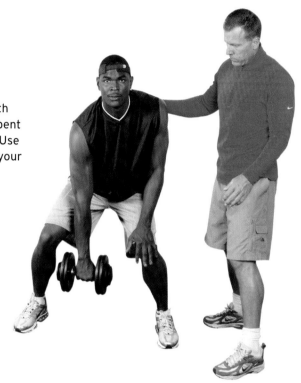

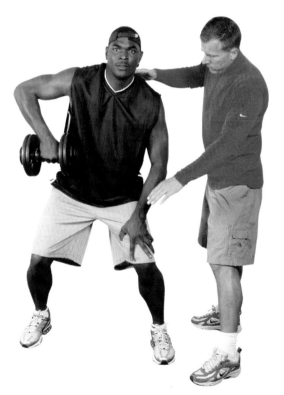

2. Once you are properly positioned on your starting point, quickly move the dumbbell up, using your hips and legs to propel the weight up in an explosive motion. As the dumbbell passes your waist, use your arm to complete the upward movement. Your elbow should be higher than your shoulder. The upward momentum should force you up onto your toes. Control the dumbbell down to its starting point.

QUICK TIPS
- Great for total body movement
- Your off hand can be resting on the knee or held away from the body
- Great for developing coordination, control, and explosion
- Intermediate/Advanced

25. Incline Press-Dumbbell

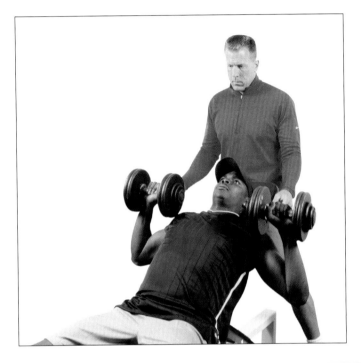

1. Hold a dumbbell in each hand, palms facing forward. The dumbbells should be resting slightly above the chest, forearms perpendicular to the floor.

2. Once the dumbbells are in a controlled position, press them up until the arms are fully extended. Hold for 2-3 seconds, then lower the dumbbells to the starting position.

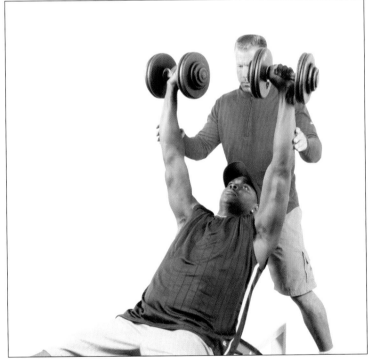

QUICK TIPS
• Use a 45-degree incline
• Always keep your buttocks on the bench
• Rest the dumbbells on your thighs before you begin the lift

26. Lateral Raise–Dumbbell

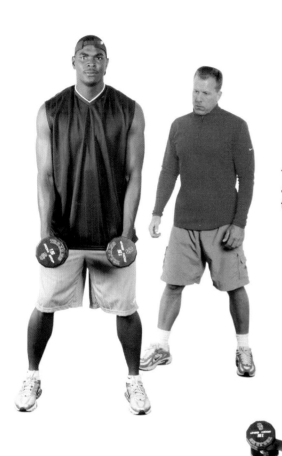

1. Stand erect with your feet shoulder-width apart. Hold the dumbbells at waist level with the arms slightly bent.

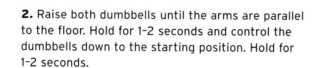

2. Raise both dumbbells until the arms are parallel to the floor. Hold for 1-2 seconds and control the dumbbells down to the starting position. Hold for 1-2 seconds.

QUICK TIPS
• Great exercise to strengthen the medial deltoids

27. Lunges–Barbell or Body Weight

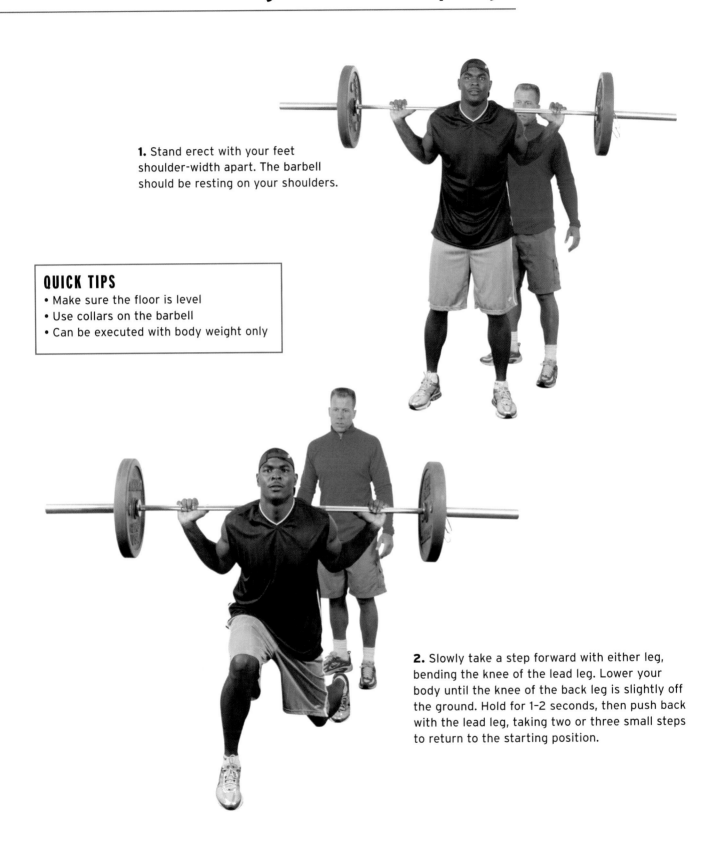

1. Stand erect with your feet shoulder-width apart. The barbell should be resting on your shoulders.

QUICK TIPS
• Make sure the floor is level
• Use collars on the barbell
• Can be executed with body weight only

2. Slowly take a step forward with either leg, bending the knee of the lead leg. Lower your body until the knee of the back leg is slightly off the ground. Hold for 1-2 seconds, then push back with the lead leg, taking two or three small steps to return to the starting position.

28. Lunges–Dumbbell

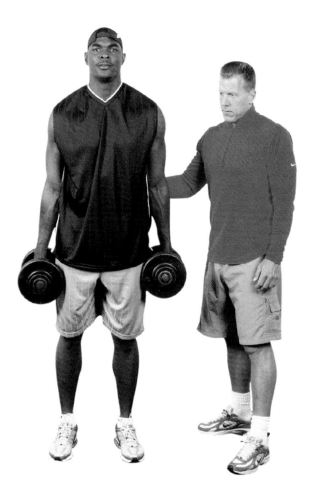

1. Stand erect with your feet shoulder-width apart. Hold the dumbbells at your sides.

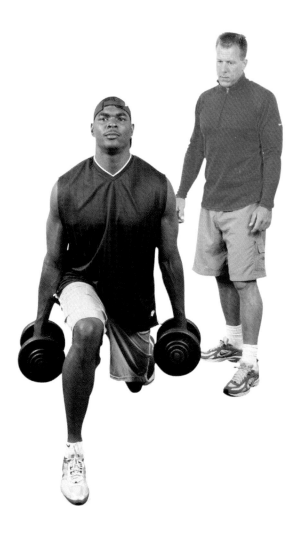

2. Slowly take a step forward with either leg, bending the knee of the lead leg. Lower your body until the knee of the back leg is slightly off the ground. Hold for 1–2 seconds, then push back with the lead leg, taking two or three small steps to return to the starting position.

QUICK TIPS
• Make sure the floor is level
• Keep the dumbbells from swinging

FW

29. Military Press–Dumbbell

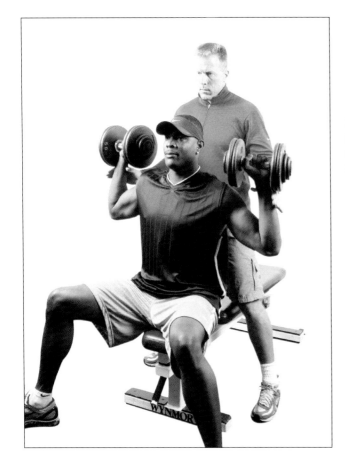

1. Hold the dumbbells slightly above the shoulders, keeping your feet flat on the floor and back straight. Balance the dumbbells before you begin the press.

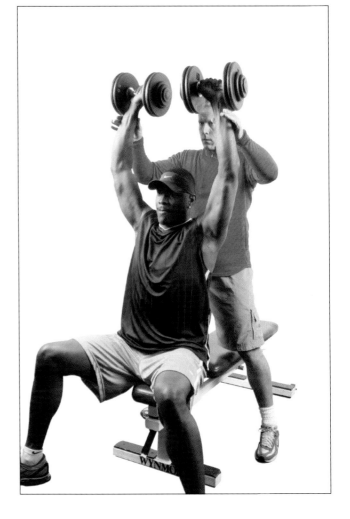

2. Once the dumbbells are balanced, push them in a straight line above your head. When your arms are fully extended, hold for 2-3 seconds. Control the dumbbells down to the starting point.

QUICK TIPS
• Keep your back straight
• Use a spotter

30. Pullovers-Dumbbell

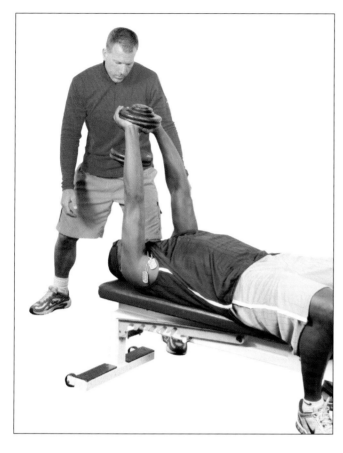

1. Position yourself flat on a bench with your feet firmly planted on the ground. With your arms extended, hold the upper end of the dumbbell in your fingers with a triangle grip.

2. Slowly move the dumbbell over your head until the lower end gently touches the floor. The dumbbell should always be about 6 inches above the face and head. After the dumbbell touches the floor, slowly pull it up to the starting position. Keep your elbows bent on the down and up movements. Once the weight plates touch the floor, slowly move the dumbbell back to the starting position. Keep the dumbbell away from your head.

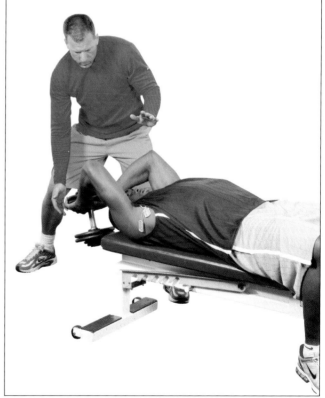

QUICK TIPS
• Use only fixed dumbbells
• Great for shoulder flexibility
• To limit the range of motion of the pull, place something on the floor behind you as a stopper

FW

31. Pullovers–Towel

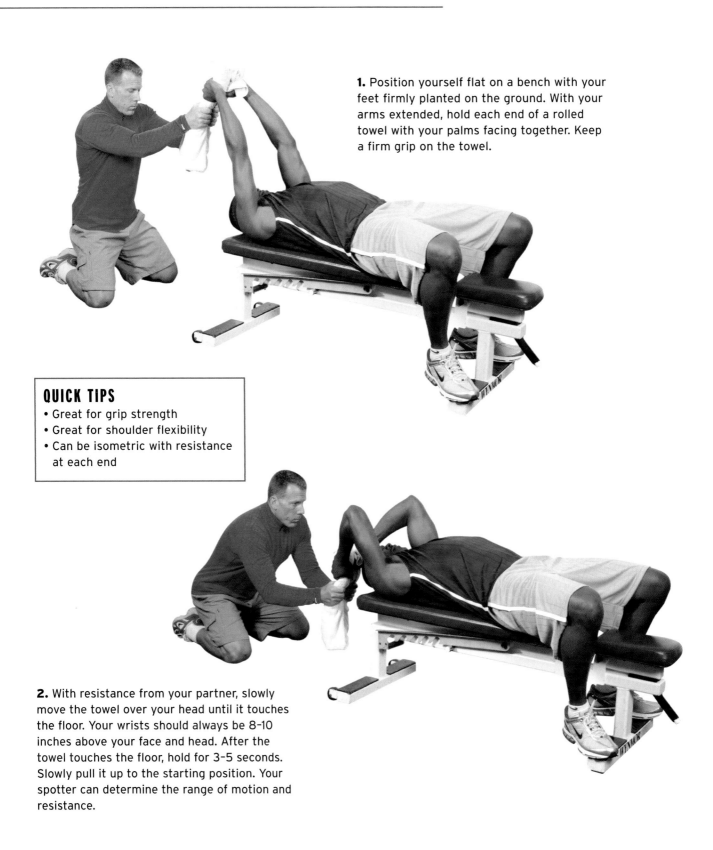

1. Position yourself flat on a bench with your feet firmly planted on the ground. With your arms extended, hold each end of a rolled towel with your palms facing together. Keep a firm grip on the towel.

QUICK TIPS
• Great for grip strength
• Great for shoulder flexibility
• Can be isometric with resistance at each end

2. With resistance from your partner, slowly move the towel over your head until it touches the floor. Your wrists should always be 8-10 inches above your face and head. After the towel touches the floor, hold for 3-5 seconds. Slowly pull it up to the starting position. Your spotter can determine the range of motion and resistance.

32. Push Press-Dumbbell

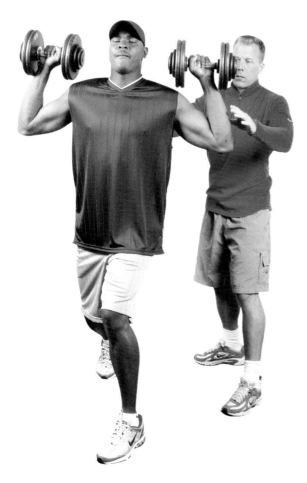

1. The push press can be completed with a split stance or a parallel, shoulder-width stance. The dumbbells should be resting at shoulder level at shoulder-width.

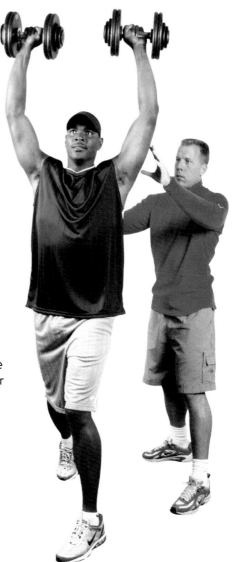

2. Once the dumbbells are stabilized, bend the knees and hips slightly and quickly extend them, pushing the dumbbells above your head. Hold the dumbbells in that position for 2-3 seconds. Lower the dumbbells in a controlled manner to the starting point.

QUICK TIPS
• Alternate the lead foot from set to set
• Find a comfortable stance before you begin
• Use your legs to move the weight

FW

33. Rice Grabs

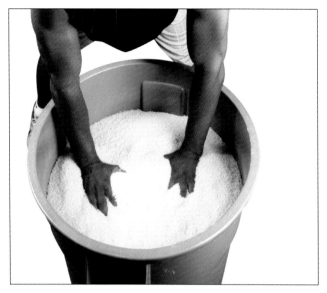

1. Stationary Open Grip: Place both hands on top of the rice. Fingers should be wide apart. Once your hands are set, quickly close and open your hands, squeezing the rice.

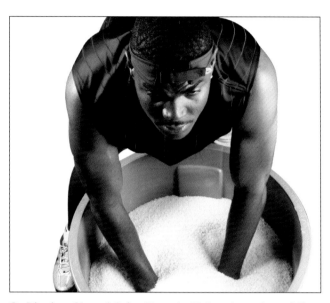

2. Digging Closed Grip: Place both hands on top of the rice with a closed grip (making a fist). Push and rotate your hands down until the rice is just below your elbows and return to the start.

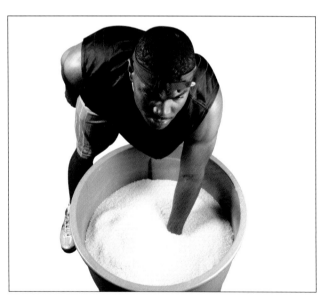

3. Digging Open Grip: Place your hand on top of the rice with fingers wide apart.

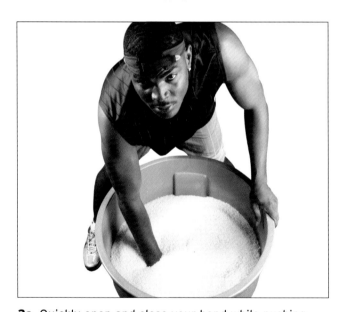

3a. Quickly open and close your hand while pushing down until the rice is just below your elbow. Do the same exercise with both hands.

QUICK TIPS
- Great for grip strength and endurance
- For greater difficulty, have a spotter hold your legs up while you do these same exercises

34. Row-Dumbbell

1. Use a bench to keep your back straight from the hips to the shoulders. Use a closed grip. Your arm should be completely straight.

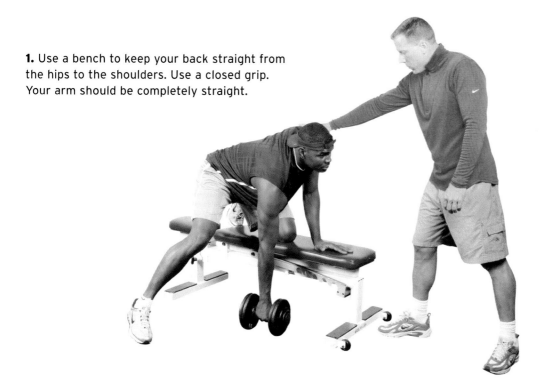

QUICK TIPS
• Keep your head in an upright position
• Your legs and back should not be used to initiate the movement

2. Pull the dumbbell up until it touches the chest area. Your elbows should be above your back at the end of the movement. Control the dumbbell down to the starting position. The knee should be slightly bent.

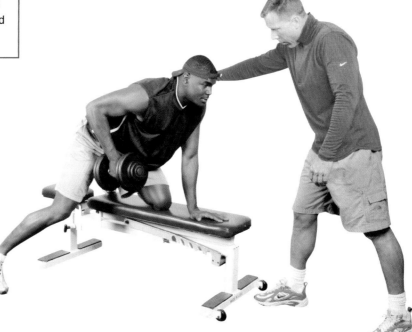

FW

35. Shoulder Shrugs–Barbell

1. Stand erect with your feet shoulder-width apart. Your arms should be completely extended with the barbell at waist level.

2. Keeping your arms straight, shrug the shoulders as high as possible. Pause at the top of the lift for 2-3 seconds. Slowly lower the weight to the starting position.

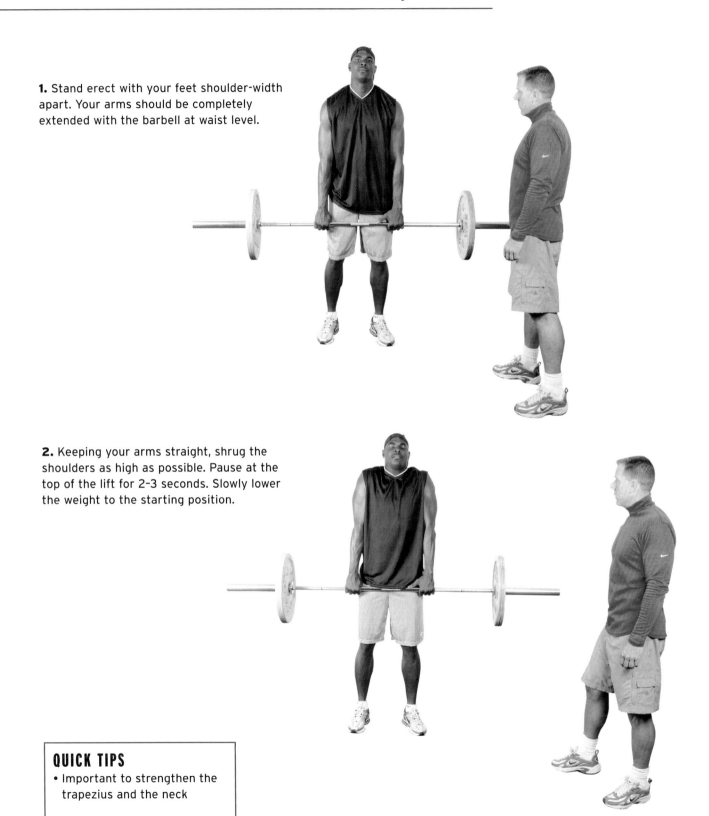

QUICK TIPS
- Important to strengthen the trapezius and the neck

36. Shoulder Shrugs-Dumbbell

1. Stand erect with your feet shoulder-width apart. Your arms should be completely extended with the dumbbells at waist level. Dumbbells are a great way to assist with grip strength.

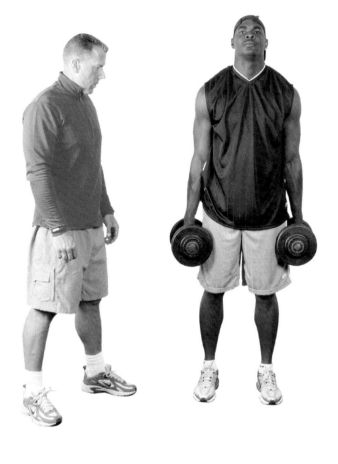

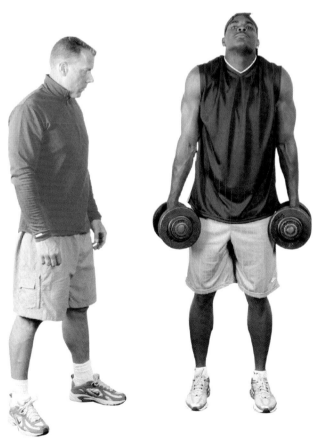

2. Keeping your arms straight, shrug the shoulders as high as possible. Pause at the top of the lift for 2-3 seconds. Slowly lower the dumbbells to the starting position.

FW

37. Squats—Barbell or Body Weight

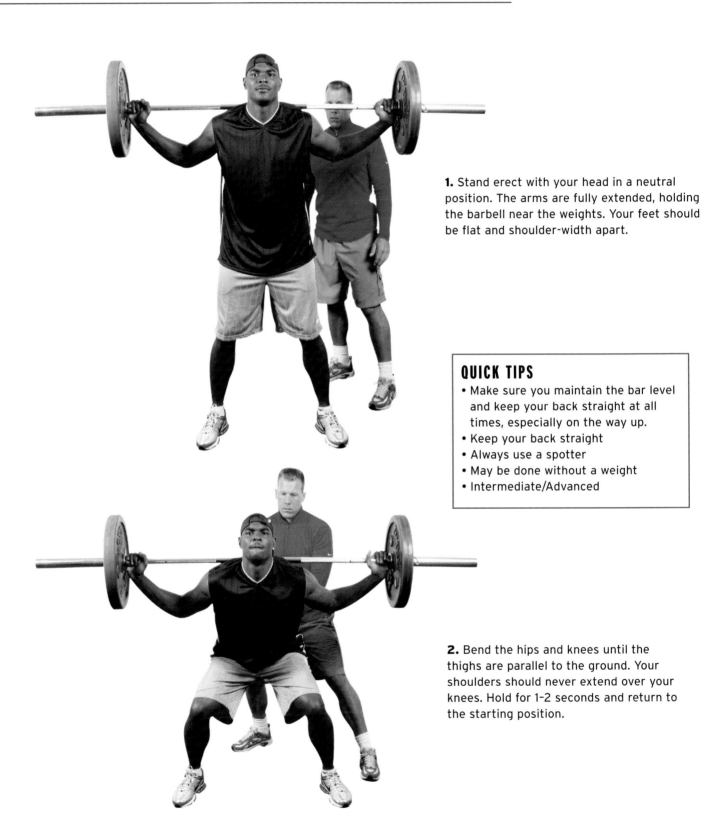

1. Stand erect with your head in a neutral position. The arms are fully extended, holding the barbell near the weights. Your feet should be flat and shoulder-width apart.

QUICK TIPS
- Make sure you maintain the bar level and keep your back straight at all times, especially on the way up.
- Keep your back straight
- Always use a spotter
- May be done without a weight
- Intermediate/Advanced

2. Bend the hips and knees until the thighs are parallel to the ground. Your shoulders should never extend over your knees. Hold for 1-2 seconds and return to the starting position.

38. Squats–Dumbbell

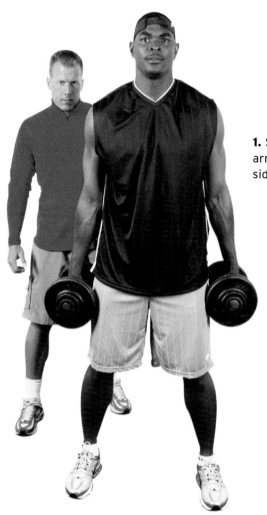

1. Stand erect with your head in a neutral position. The arms are fully extended, holding the dumbbells at your sides. Your feet should be flat and shoulder-width apart.

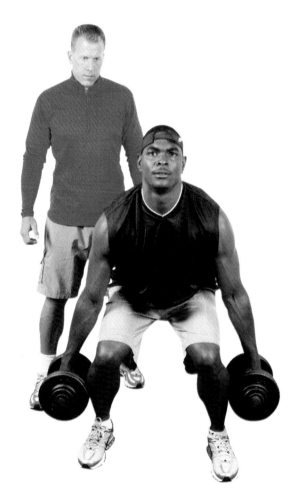

2. Bend the hips and knees until the thighs are parallel to the ground. Your shoulders should never extend over your knees. Hold for 1-2 seconds and return to the starting position.

QUICK TIPS
• Good lift for beginners

FW

39. Straight-Leg Dead Lifts–Barbell

1. Stand erect with your feet shoulder-width apart. Your arms should be completely extended while holding the weight at waist level. Keep your knees slightly bent.

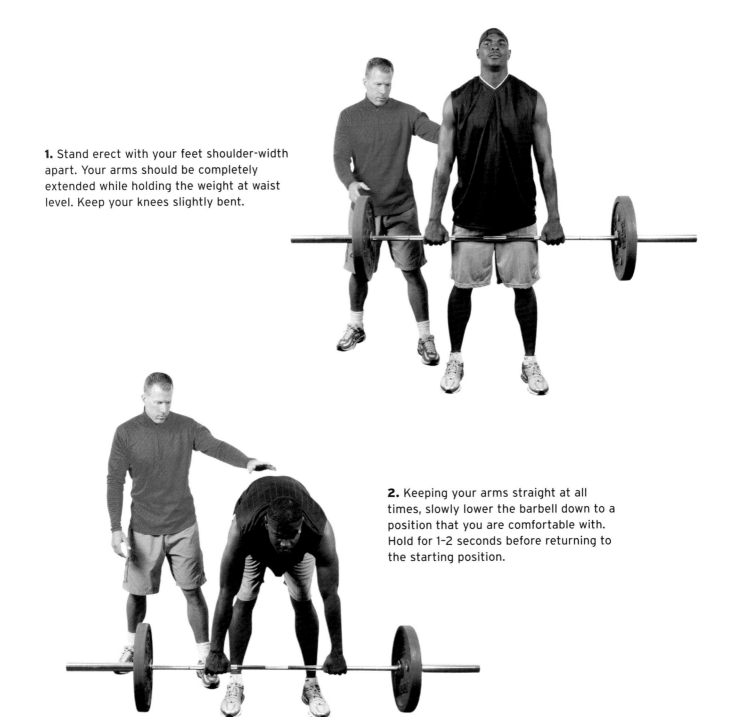

2. Keeping your arms straight at all times, slowly lower the barbell down to a position that you are comfortable with. Hold for 1-2 seconds before returning to the starting position.

QUICK TIPS
- Advanced: Use a platform to increase range of motion

40. Straight-Leg Dead Lifts–Dumbbell

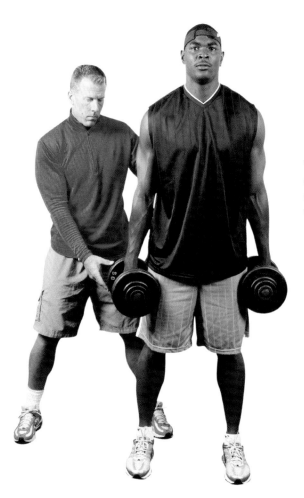

1. Stand erect with your feet shoulder-width apart. Your arms should be completely extended while holding the dumbbells at waist level. Keep your knees slightly bent.

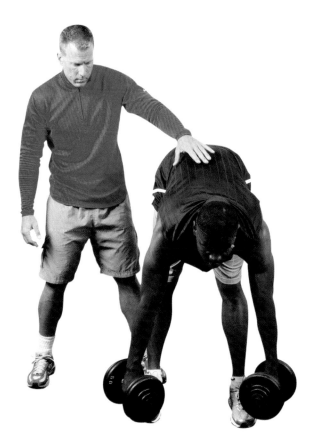

2. Keeping your arms straight at all times, slowly lower the dumbbells down to a position that you are comfortable with. Hold for 1–2 seconds before returning to the starting position.

QUICK TIPS
• Advanced: Use a platform to increase the range of motion

FW

41. Upright Row–Barbell/Dumbbell/Plate

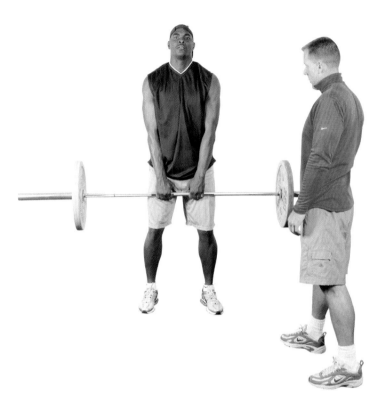

1. Stand erect with feet shoulder-width apart. Your palms should face your body with your hands 6-8 inches apart. Make sure the barbell is balanced, your arms are fully extend, and your knees are slightly bent.

2. Pull the weight up toward your chin. The up movement should terminate approximately at your collarbone, elbows higher than your shoulders. Lower the weight in a controlled manner to the starting point.

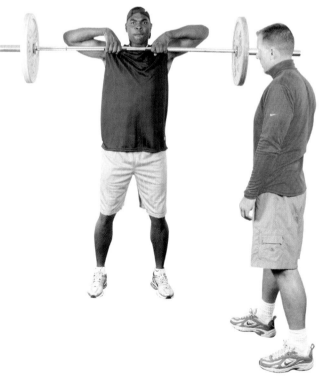

QUICK TIPS
• Great lift for beginners and a great way to develop finger and grip strength
• Keep your head in an upright position
• Your legs and back should not be used to initiate the movement
• Intermediate/Advanced: Use dumbbells or plate. Dumbbells give you a great technique for determining your dominant side

42. Curls-Dumbbell

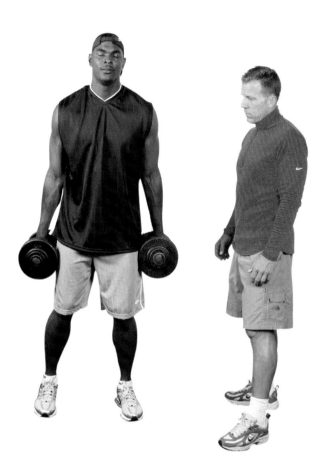

1. Use a parallel stance with your legs slightly bent and hold the dumbbells at your side.

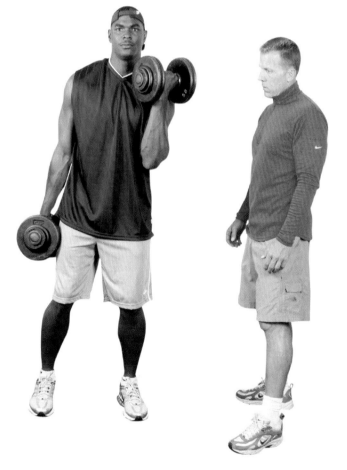

2. In a controlled manner, move your arm upward to a flexed position.

QUICK TIPS
• You can alternate arms or repeat one side and then do the other

FW

43. Curls–Towel

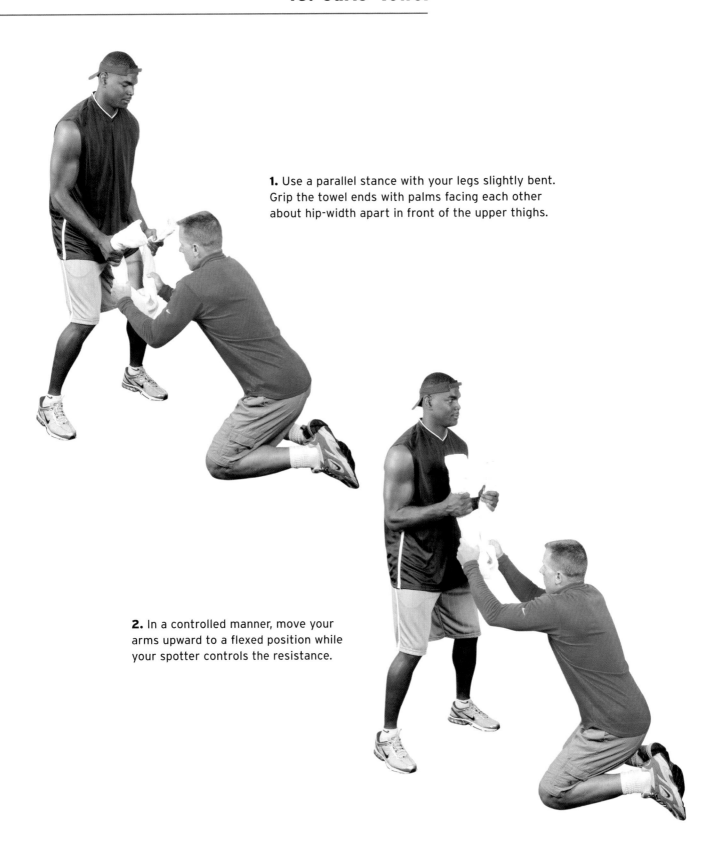

1. Use a parallel stance with your legs slightly bent. Grip the towel ends with palms facing each other about hip-width apart in front of the upper thighs.

2. In a controlled manner, move your arms upward to a flexed position while your spotter controls the resistance.

44. Power Clean-Barbell

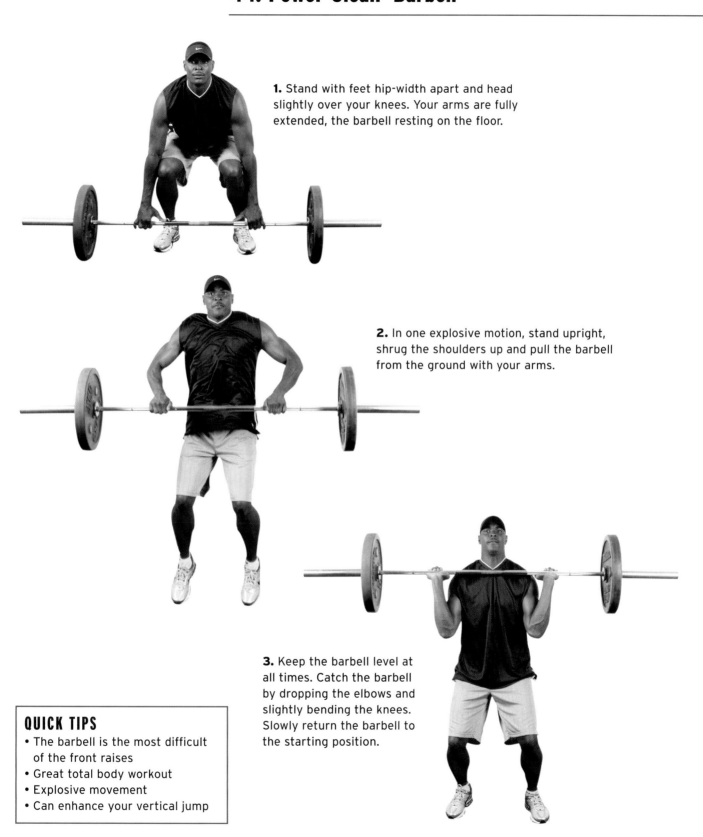

1. Stand with feet hip-width apart and head slightly over your knees. Your arms are fully extended, the barbell resting on the floor.

2. In one explosive motion, stand upright, shrug the shoulders up and pull the barbell from the ground with your arms.

3. Keep the barbell level at all times. Catch the barbell by dropping the elbows and slightly bending the knees. Slowly return the barbell to the starting position.

QUICK TIPS
- The barbell is the most difficult of the front raises
- Great total body workout
- Explosive movement
- Can enhance your vertical jump

FW

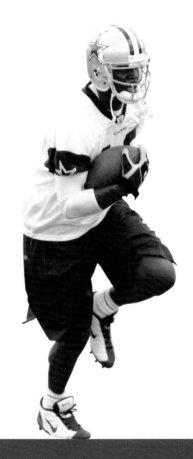

ISOLATERALS

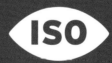

45. Bench Press-Isolateral

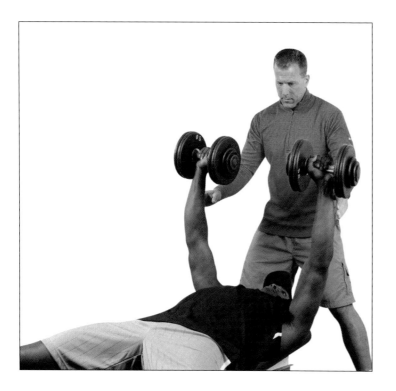

1. Hold a dumbbell in each hand, palms facing forward. Keep a solid base with your feet flat on the ground. Keep one arm extended while your opposite arm is working.

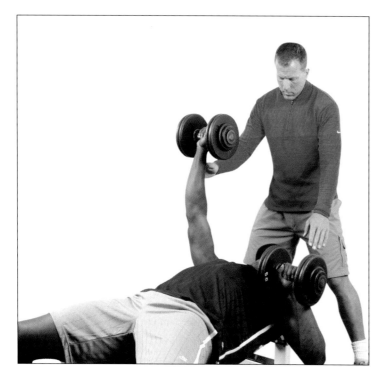

2. While holding one dumbbell at the starting point, slowly lower the other until it touches the outside of the chest. Once it touches, push it back to the starting point.

QUICK TIPS
- Do all reps on one side, then do reps on the other for each set as explained above
- Intermediate/Advanced

46. Front Raise-Isolateral

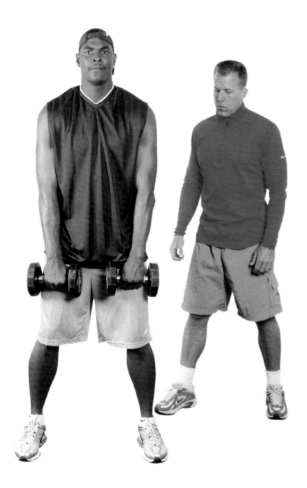

1. Stand erect with feet approximately shoulder-width apart, holding a dumbbell in each hand. Work one side at a time.

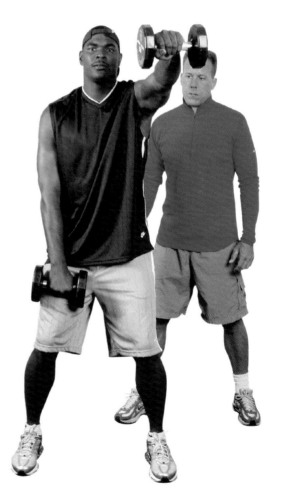

2. Raise one dumbbell to eye level. Hold for 1-2 seconds at the top, then slowly return to the starting position.

QUICK TIPS
• Great exercise to strengthen the anterior deltoid

ISO

47. Incline Press-Isolateral

1. Hold a dumbbell in each hand, palms facing forward. Keep a solid base with your feet flat on the ground. Keep one arm extended while the opposite arm is working.

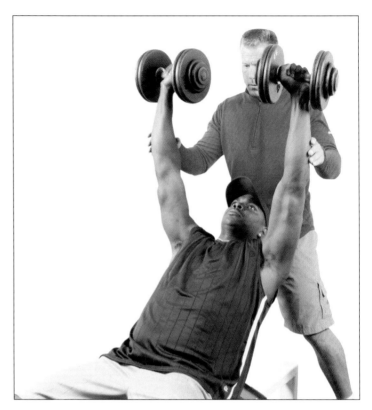

2. While holding one dumbbell at the starting point, slowly lower the other side until the dumbbell is slightly above the upper chest area. At this point, press it back to the starting position.

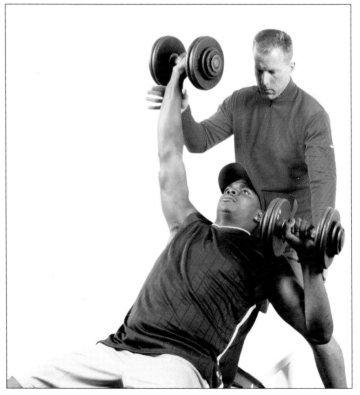

QUICK TIPS
• Intermediate/Advanced

48. Lateral Raise-Isolateral

1. Stand erect with your feet shoulder-width apart. Hold the dumbbells at waist level with the arms slightly bent. Raise one of the dumbbells until the arm is parallel to the floor.

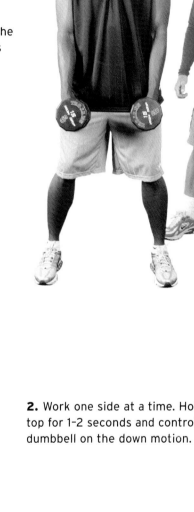

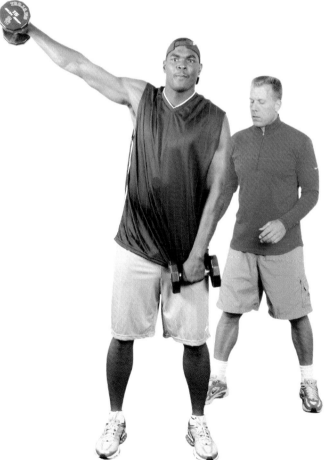

2. Work one side at a time. Hold at the top for 1-2 seconds and control the dumbbell on the down motion.

QUICK TIPS
- Work one side at a time
- Great for muscular balance

ISO

49. Military Press–Isolateral

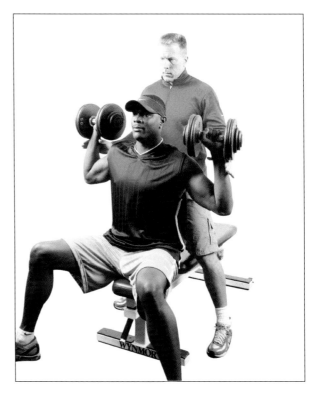

1. Hold the dumbbells slightly above the shoulders, keeping your feet flat on the floor and back straight. Balance the dumbbells before you begin the press.

2. Once the dumbbells are balanced, push one in a straight line above your head. When your arm is fully extended, hold for 2-3 seconds. Control the dumbbell down to the starting point. Balance the dumbbells and repeat with opposite arm.

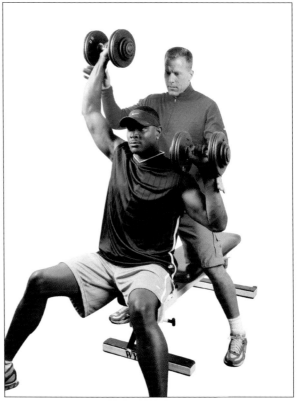

QUICK TIPS
- Find a balance point
- Use a spotter
- Intermediate/Advanced

50. Push Press-Isolateral

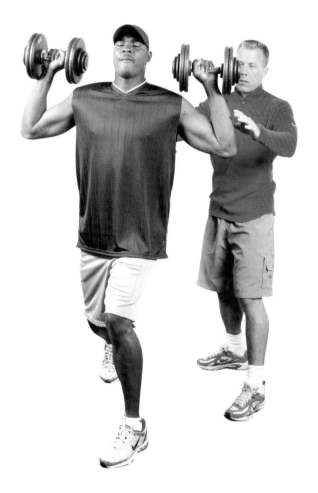

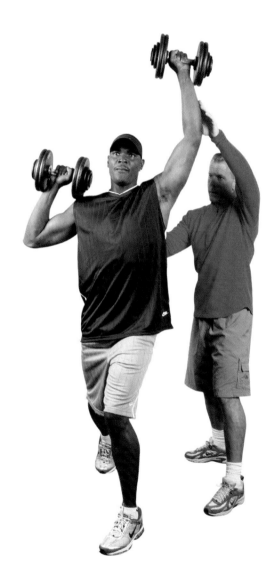

1. The push press can be completed with a split stance or a parallel shoulder-width stance. The dumbbells should be resting at shoulder level and shoulder-width.

2. Once the dumbbells are stabilized, bend the knees and hips slightly and quickly extend one arm, pushing one dumbbell above your head while holding the other at chest level. Hold the dumbbell in that position for 2-3 seconds. Lower the dumbbell in a controlled manner to the starting point. After one set, switch and do the other side.

QUICK TIPS
• Alternate the lead foot with each set
• Know your dominant side so you work the opposite side to balance your muscles
• Use a spotter
• Intermediate/Advanced

ISO

51. Upright Row-Isolateral

1. Stand erect with feet shoulder-width apart. Grip the dumbbells with palms facing your body and hands 6–8 inches apart. Make sure the dumbbells are balanced and your arms are fully extended. Pull the weight up toward your chin.

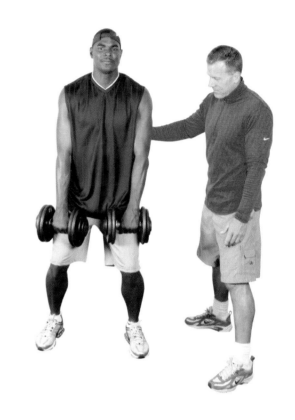

QUICK TIPS
• Can be done by beginners as well as advanced lifters
• Great way to develop strength on your nondominant side

2. Work one side at a time. The upward movement should terminate approximately at your collarbone. Lower the weight in a controlled manner to the starting point.

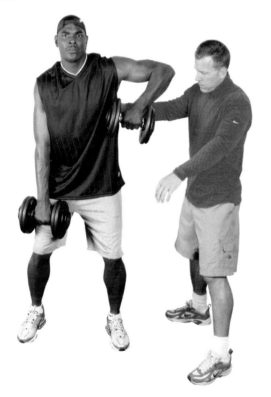

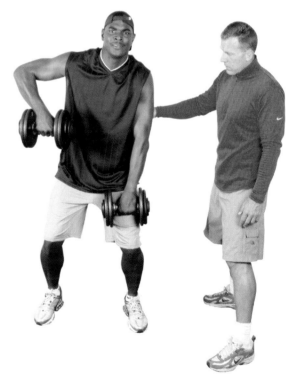

52. Leg Press–Isolateral

1. Seated on a leg press machine, position your feet and legs to your comfort.

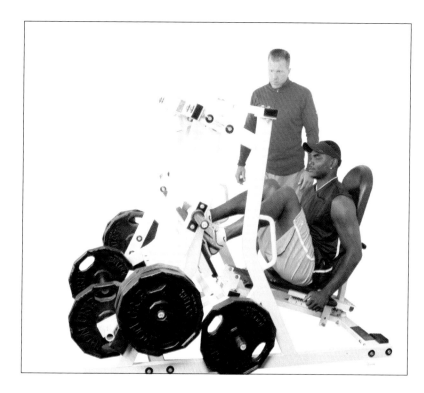

2. Once you are positioned comfortably, in a controlled motion push one of your feet outward, extending the leg. Always keep your body on the seat and never "lock" your knee at the end of the movement. Control the weights on the way down as well.

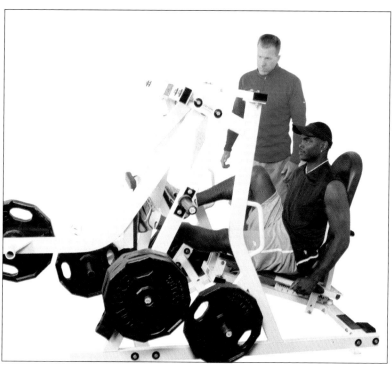

QUICK TIPS
- Work both legs
- You may do all sets on one side or alternate legs

ISO

53. Leg Extension-Isolateral

1. Seated on a leg extension machine, make sure the pads are positioned slightly above the top of your feet.

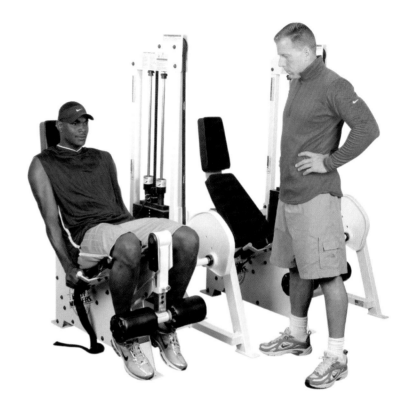

2. Once you are correctly positioned, extend your leg upward. Lower to starting position. Both movements should always be controlled.

QUICK TIPS
• Do all the repetitions to one leg and then work the other leg

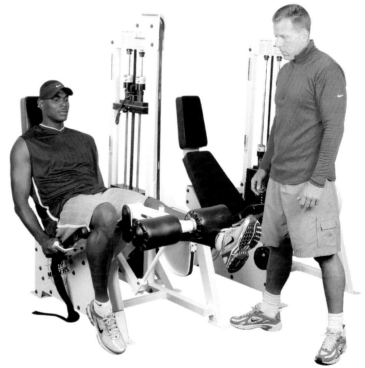

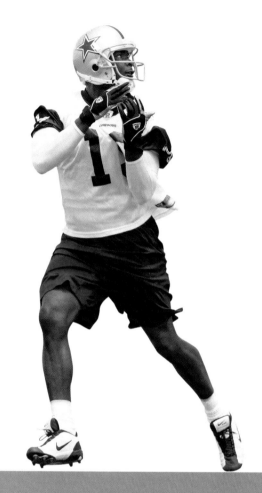

MACHINE EXERCISES

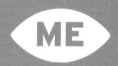

54. Pull-Downs–Wide Grip

1. Seated on a pull-down machine, reach upward and grab the bar using a wide grip. Your arms should be fully extended.

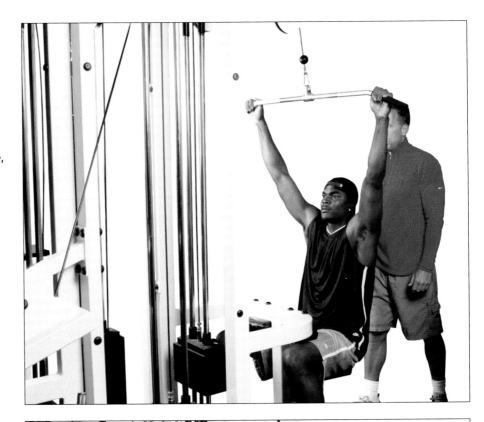

2. In a controlled manner, pull the bar downward. Pull the bar just below your chin and slowly return the bar up to the starting point.

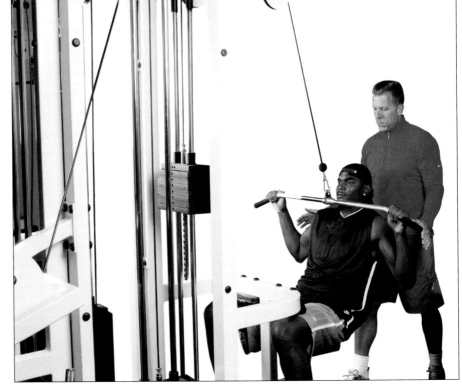

55. Pull-Downs–Reverse Grip

1. Seated on a pull-down machine, reach upward and grab the bar using a reverse grip. Your arms should be fully extended.

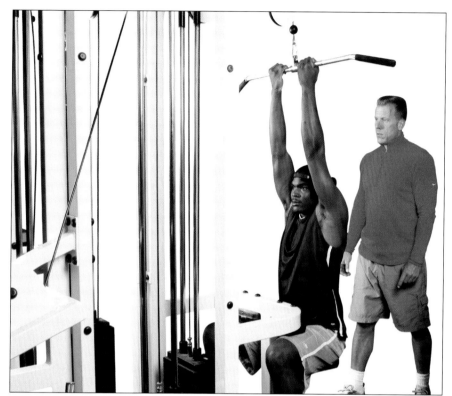

2. In a controlled manner, pull the bar downward. Pull the bar just below your chin and slowly return the bar up to the starting point.

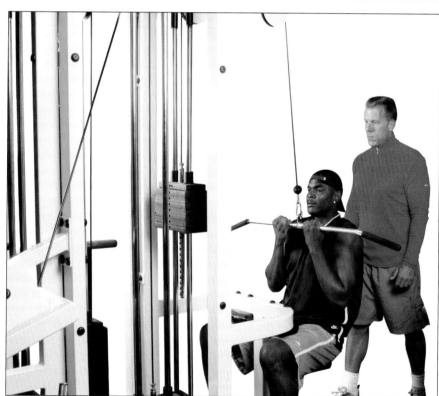

ME

56. Leg Extension

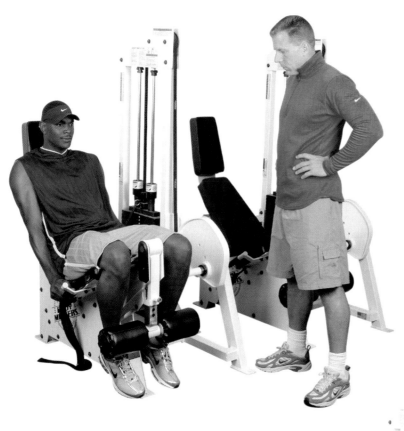

1. Seated on a leg extension machine, make sure the pads are positioned slightly above the top of your feet.

2. Once you are correctly positioned, extend your legs upward. Lower to the starting position. Both movements should always be in a controlled manner.

57. Leg Flexion

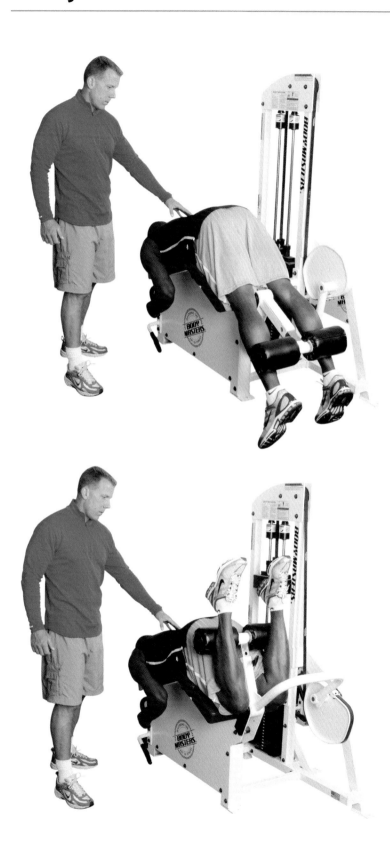

1. Lie on a flex machine. Position the pads slightly below your calves.

2. Once you are in position, curl or flex your legs upward. The movement should always be in a controlled manner. Slowly lower to starting position.

ME

58. Leg Press

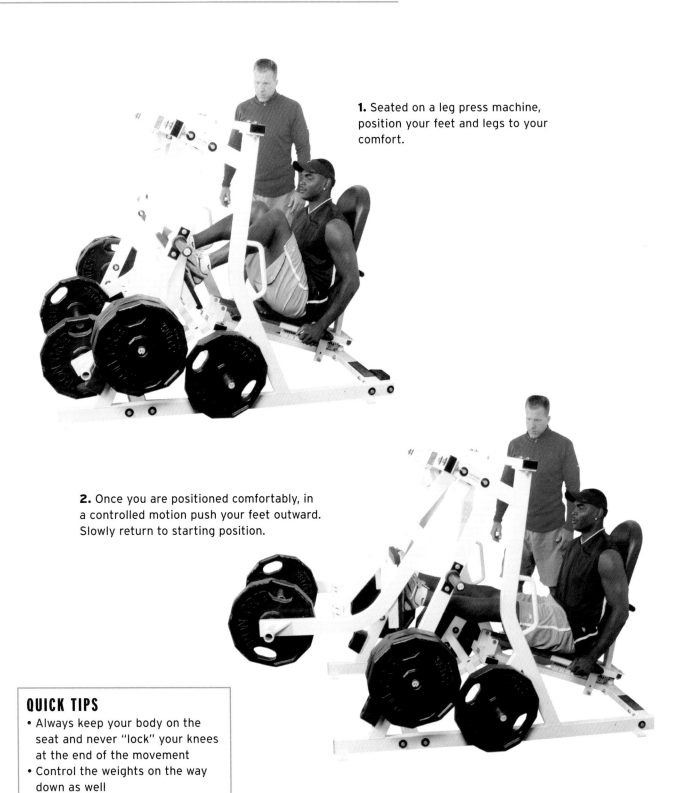

1. Seated on a leg press machine, position your feet and legs to your comfort.

2. Once you are positioned comfortably, in a controlled motion push your feet outward. Slowly return to starting position.

QUICK TIPS
- Always keep your body on the seat and never "lock" your knees at the end of the movement
- Control the weights on the way down as well

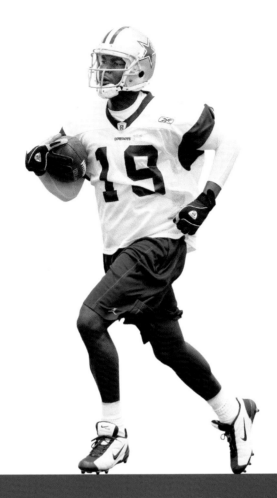

PLYOMETRICS

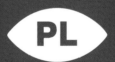

59a. Box Jumps–Small Box

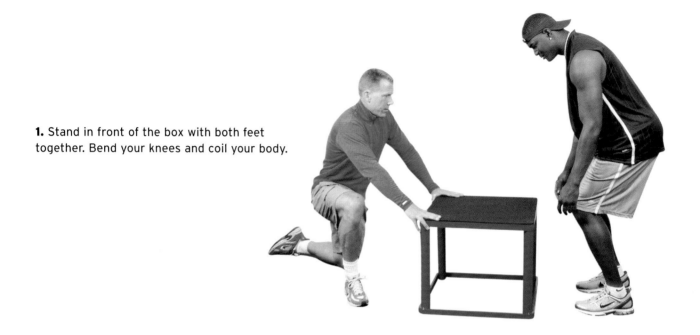

1. Stand in front of the box with both feet together. Bend your knees and coil your body.

2. Pushing off your legs, do an explosive jump up to the top of the box. Jump back down to the start position.

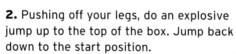

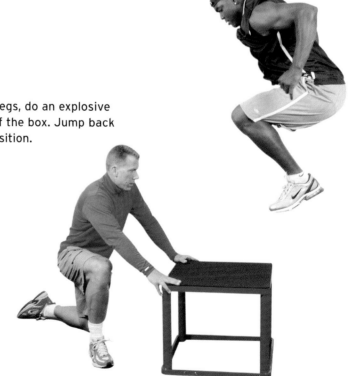

QUICK TIPS
- Make sure the box is steady
- Start with a box that is not too high so you can accomplish the jump
- Be careful not to miss the landing
- Land on the balls of your feet
- Bend at the knees when landing

59b. Box Jumps–Big Box

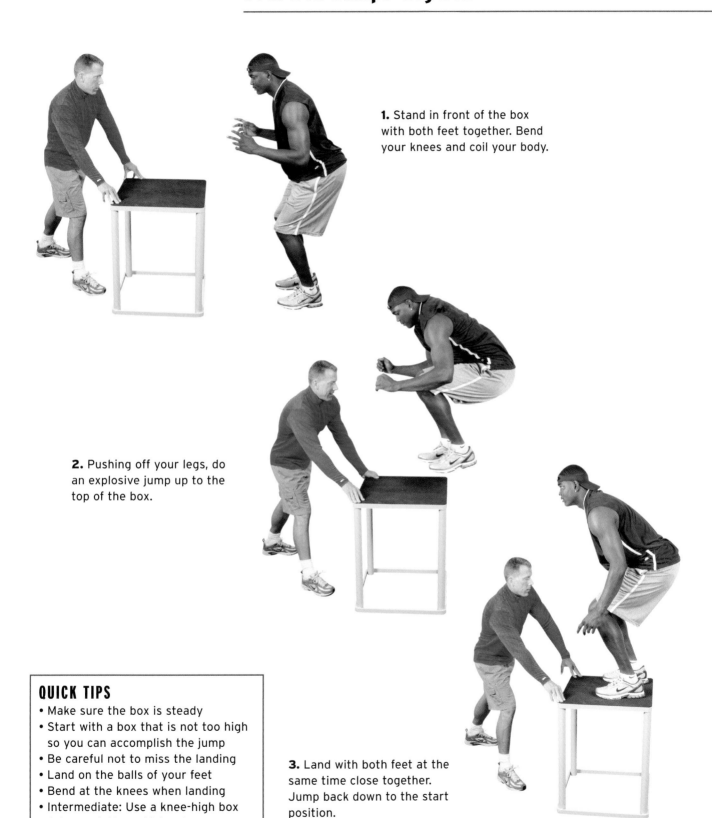

1. Stand in front of the box with both feet together. Bend your knees and coil your body.

2. Pushing off your legs, do an explosive jump up to the top of the box.

3. Land with both feet at the same time close together. Jump back down to the start position.

QUICK TIPS
- Make sure the box is steady
- Start with a box that is not too high so you can accomplish the jump
- Be careful not to miss the landing
- Land on the balls of your feet
- Bend at the knees when landing
- Intermediate: Use a knee-high box
- Advanced: Use a higher box

PL

60. Step-Ups

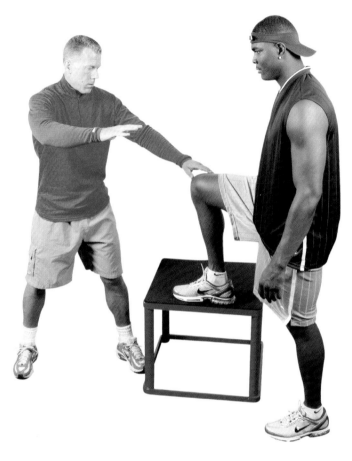

1. Stand with one foot firmly placed on top of the box. Hands should be held at waist level. Thigh is parallel to the floor.

2. With one quick motion, extend the top leg while bringing the opposite leg up to your chest. The movement should be a quick jump.

3. Return to the starting position and repeat the motion. Make sure you repeat the exercise with the other leg and work both sides equally.

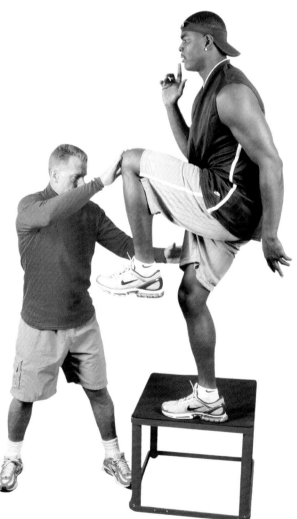

QUICK TIPS
• Great exercise to develop leg strength

61. Lateral Jumps—Long Way

1. Begin the exercise with outside foot near one of the cones. Hands should be shoulder level. The opposite leg should be slightly bent.

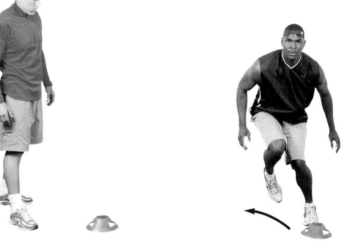

2. With a quick motion, extend the top leg while pushing off with the opposite leg.

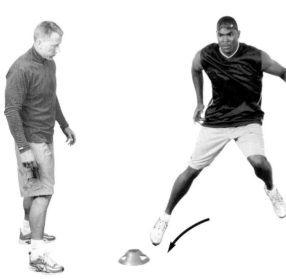

3. Once you land, repeat the motion and work both sides equally.

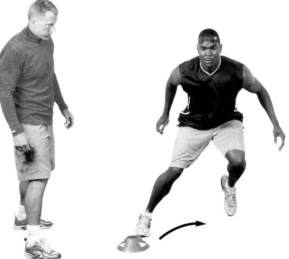

QUICK TIPS
• Great way to develop lateral movement
• Intermediate/Advanced

PL

62. Medicine Ball Ground Work—One Hand

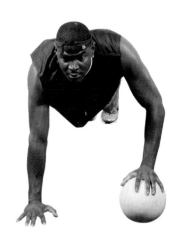

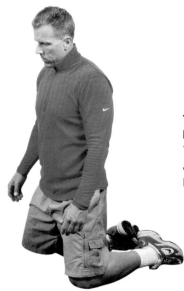

1. Start by placing one hand on the ball and the other on the ground. Your legs are wide apart and your arms slightly bent. Move your hand back and forth over the ball.

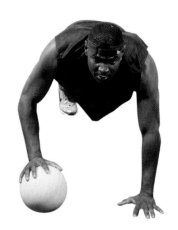

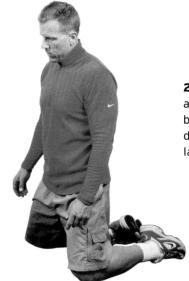

2. Quickly move one hand off the ball as the other hand comes on to the ball. Move your feet in the same direction as your hands. Use quick lateral movement over the ball.

QUICK TIPS
- Always use a spotter
- Great for upper body endurance
- Great for lateral movement and eye-body coordination
- Good upper-body plyometric exercise

63. Medicine Ball Walk/Hold/Balance

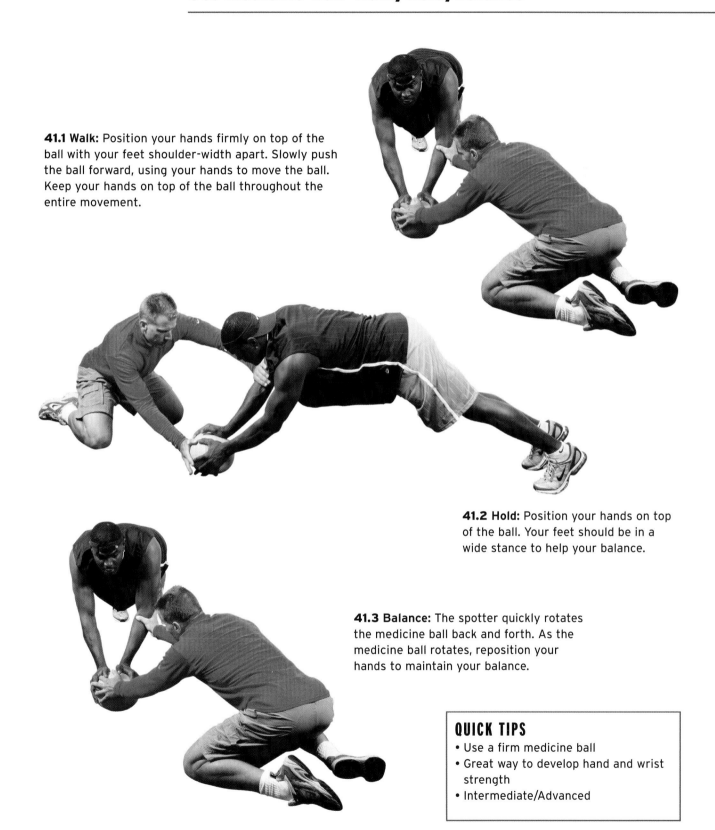

41.1 Walk: Position your hands firmly on top of the ball with your feet shoulder-width apart. Slowly push the ball forward, using your hands to move the ball. Keep your hands on top of the ball throughout the entire movement.

41.2 Hold: Position your hands on top of the ball. Your feet should be in a wide stance to help your balance.

41.3 Balance: The spotter quickly rotates the medicine ball back and forth. As the medicine ball rotates, reposition your hands to maintain your balance.

QUICK TIPS
- Use a firm medicine ball
- Great way to develop hand and wrist strength
- Intermediate/Advanced

PL

64. Push-Ups–Plyometric

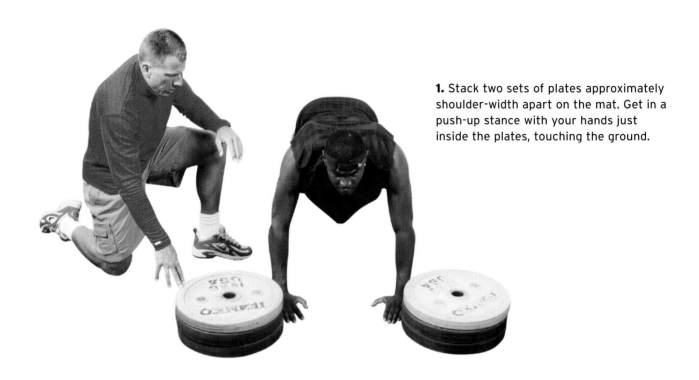

1. Stack two sets of plates approximately shoulder-width apart on the mat. Get in a push-up stance with your hands just inside the plates, touching the ground.

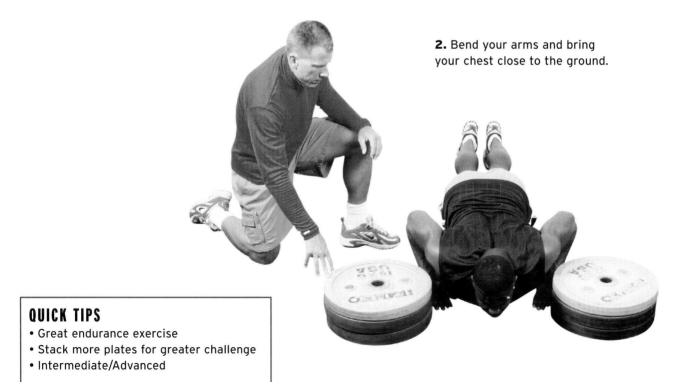

2. Bend your arms and bring your chest close to the ground.

QUICK TIPS
- Great endurance exercise
- Stack more plates for greater challenge
- Intermediate/Advanced

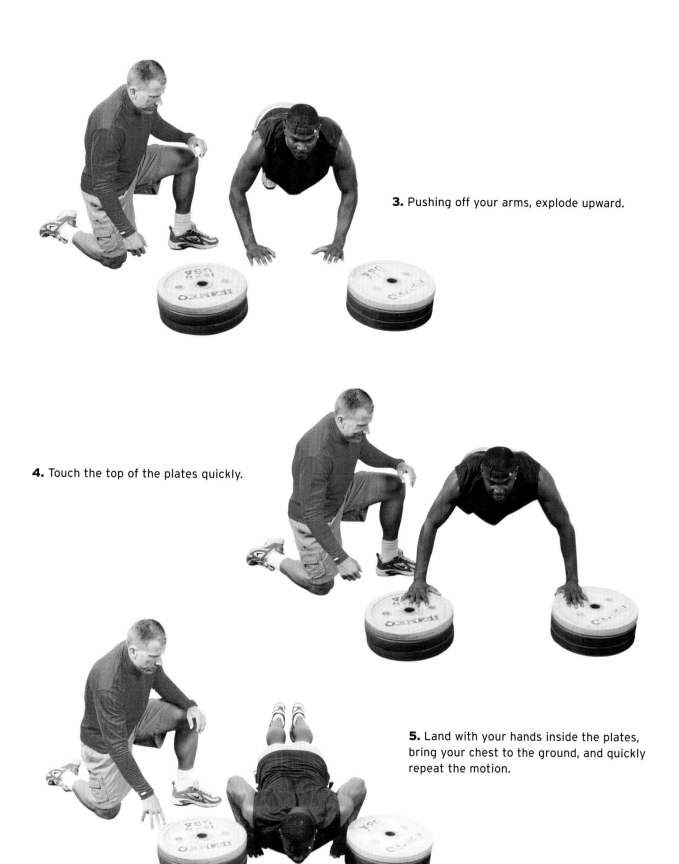

3. Pushing off your arms, explode upward.

4. Touch the top of the plates quickly.

5. Land with your hands inside the plates, bring your chest to the ground, and quickly repeat the motion.

PL

65. Bench Squat with One Leg–Body Weight

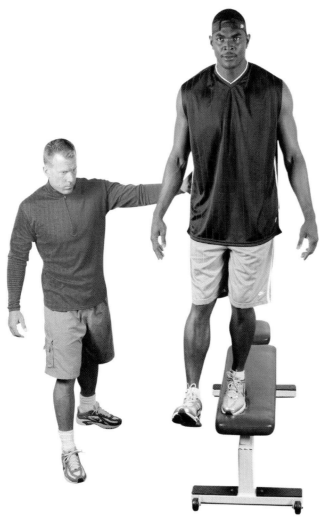

1. Standing on a box or a bench, place one foot firmly on top of the bench and let the other hang to the outside. Slightly bend your active or supporting leg to ensure your balance.

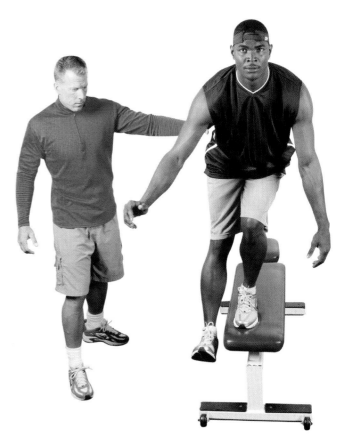

QUICK TIPS
• Make sure the bench or box is stable
• Use your arms and spotter for balance

2. Once you are positioned correctly, slowly bend your active leg as you lower your body. Bend your leg to your comfort level, then return upward to the starting position.

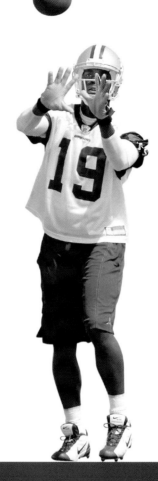

POWER SERIES

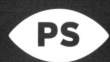

66. 3-Way Warm-Up

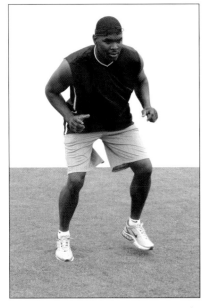
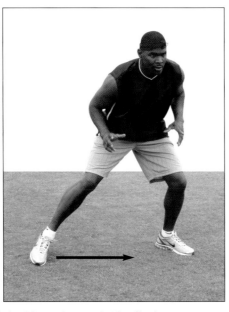
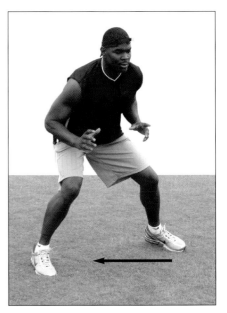

Phase 1: Place two cones approximately 40 yards apart. The first movement is a lateral shuffle. Shuffle your feet to the left, leading with your left leg, for 40 yards.

Repeat the process with your right leg, coming back for 40 yards. Total distance of the drill: 80 yards.

Phase 2: Place two cones approximately 40 yards apart. The second movement is a lateral cross-step. Run sideways from cone to cone, crossing your feet and arms. Start stepping from right to left, leading with left leg in front. Step clear across.

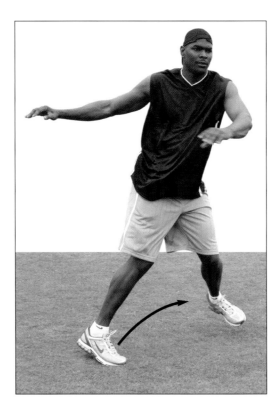
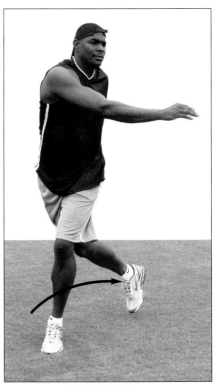

Cross-step with your right leg behind your left.

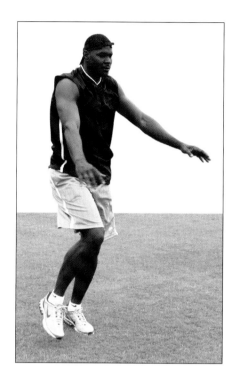 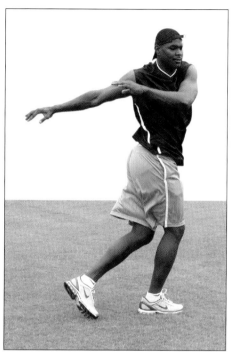

Continue cross-stepping with one leg in front and then in back. Return to your right doing the same motion. Total distance of the drill: 80 yards.

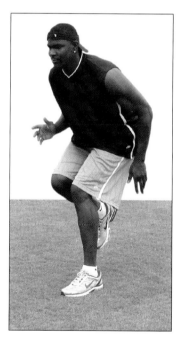 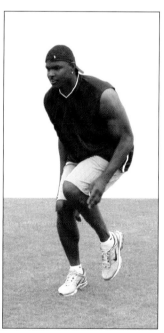 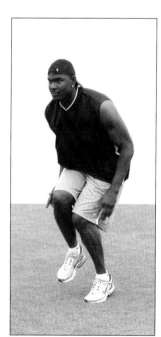 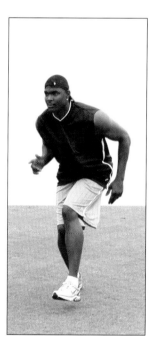

Phase 3: Follow the same 40-yard format. Backpedal 40 yards, then return to the starting point. Total distance of the drill: 80 yards.

67. 3-Cone Drill

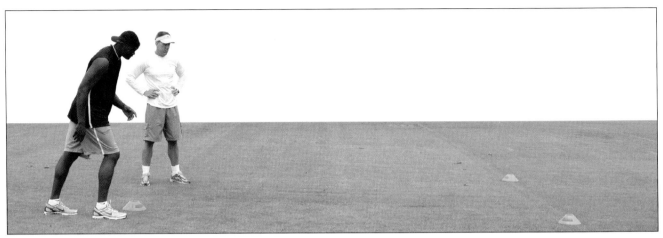

1. Start with 3 cones approximately 5 yards apart in an L-shaped format. Use a split stance to position your body.

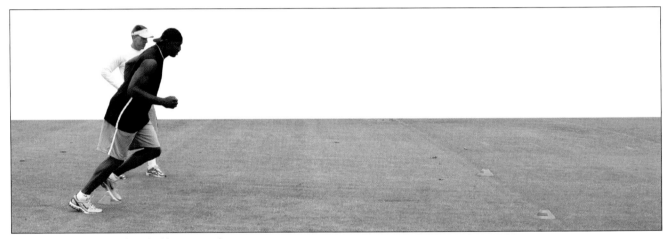

2. Run in a straight line to the second cone.

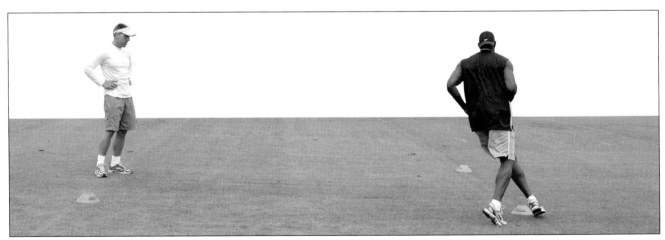

3. As your begin to accelerate, prepare to make a left turn at the second cone.

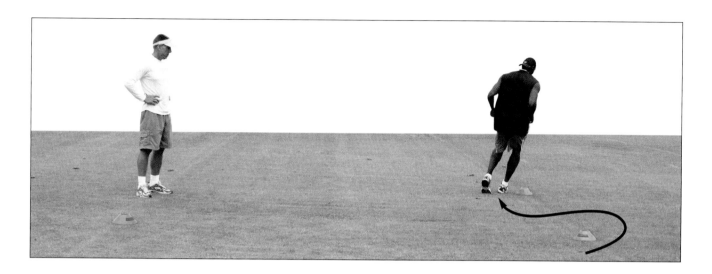

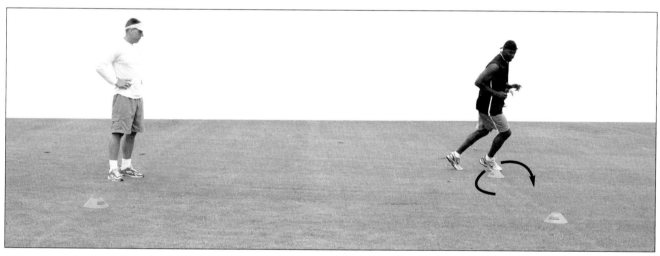

4. After you've rounded the second cone, accelerate to the third cone and make an 180-degree turn around the cone going inside in a clockwise motion.

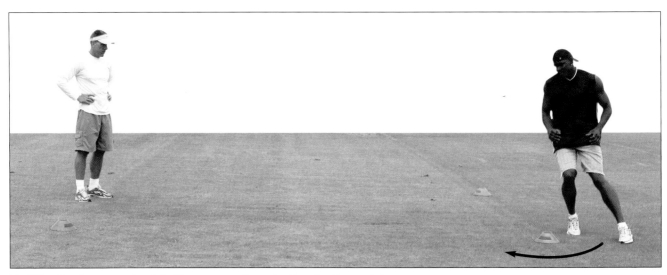

5. After the turn, run back in the same pattern to the starting point.
Accelerate back to cone 2 and prepare for the . . .

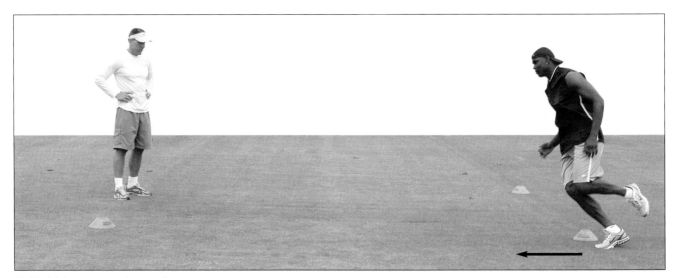

6. Right turn around cone 2 . . .

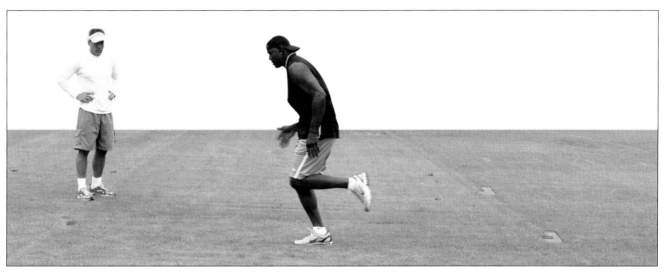

7. And accelerate to cone 1. Total distance of the drill: 20 yards.

68. 4-Cone Drill

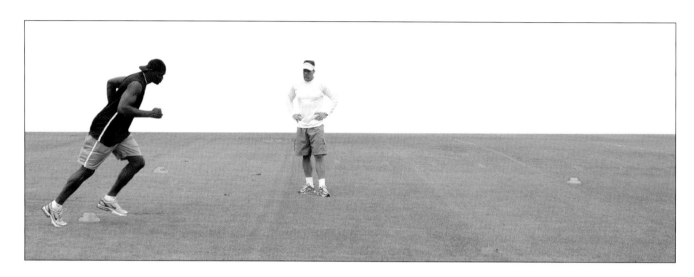

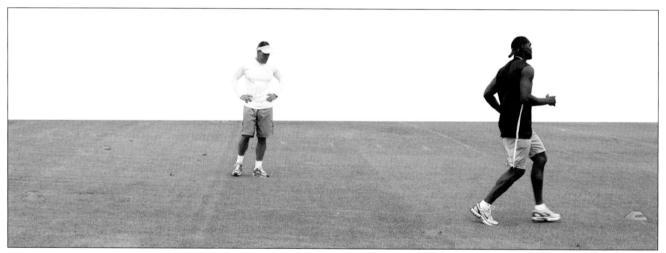

1. Start with 4 cones approximately 10 yards apart in a square formation. Begin the drill by running straight ahead to the first cone.

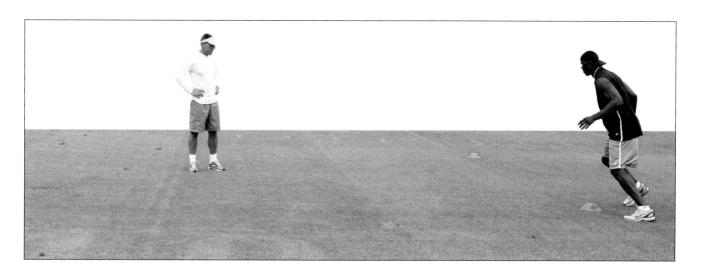

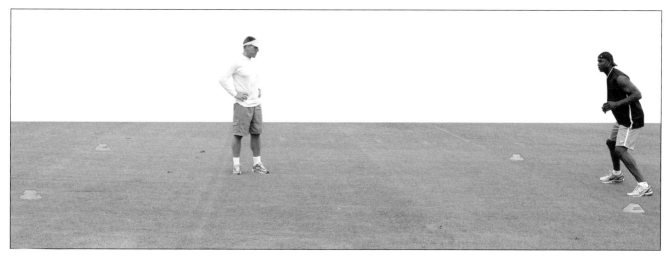

2. As you round the first cone, move to a lateral shuffle, leading with your right leg. Move quickly and with good balance.

PS

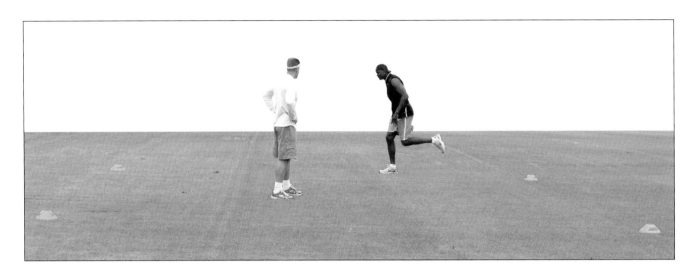

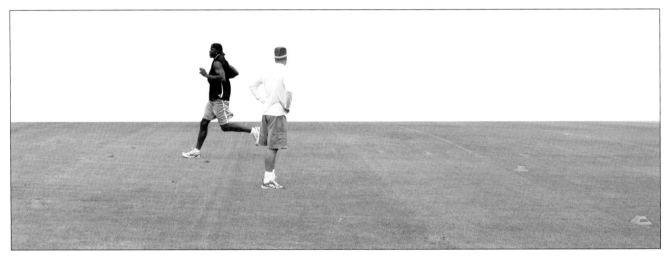

3. As you round the second cone, open into a quick forward
run. Prepare to decelerate as the third cone approaches.

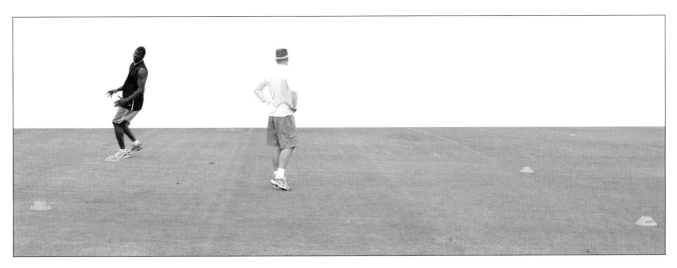

4. Round the third cone, and go back into a lateral shuffle, leading with your left leg. Pass the fourth cone to complete the drill.

69. "5 - 10 - 5" Drill

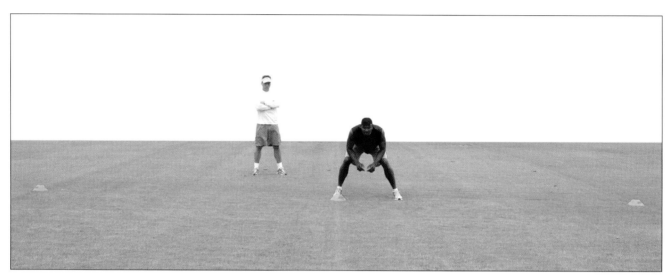

1. Place 3 cones in a straight line 5 yards apart from each other. Line up over the middle cone.

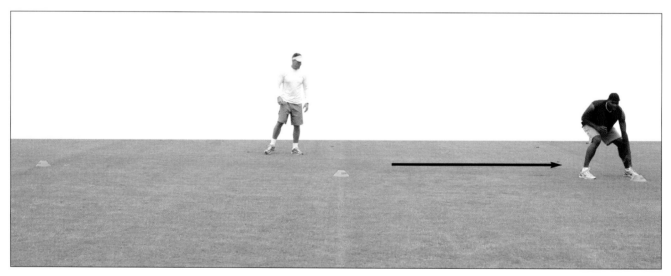

2. Once your feet are set, turn and run straight to an outside cone. Once you reach the cone, touch the top of the cone with your fingers.

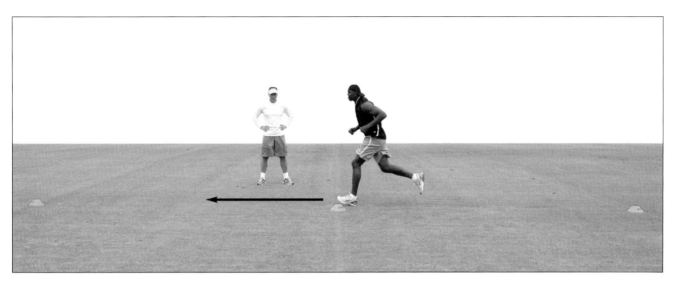

3. Redirect and accelerate to the other side.

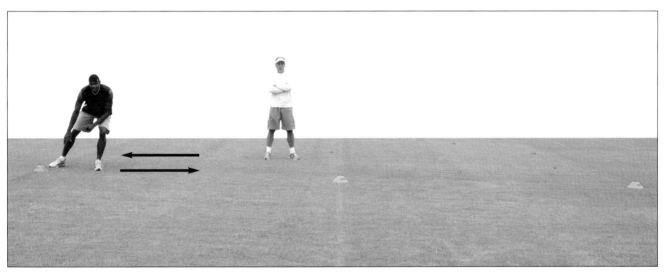

4. As you reach the outside cone, touch the tip of the cone with your fingers, redirect and run back to the middle cone. Total distance of the drill: approximately 20 yards.

70. "5 - 10" Drill

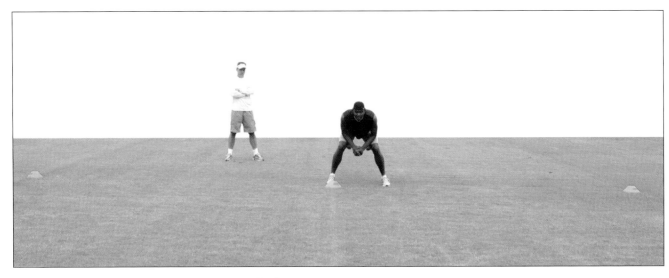

1. Place 3 cones approximately 5 yards apart. Line up over the middle cone.

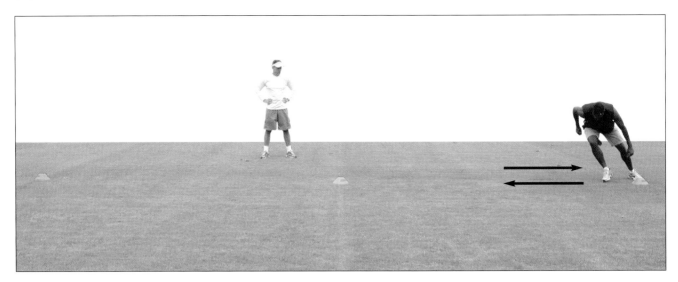

2. Once you are set and ready, turn and run to the outside cone. Touch the top of the cone.

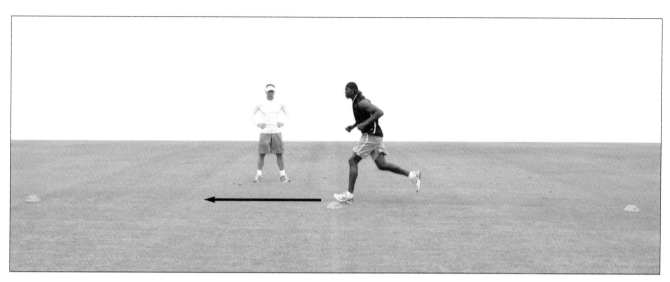

3. Redirect and accelerate to the other side.

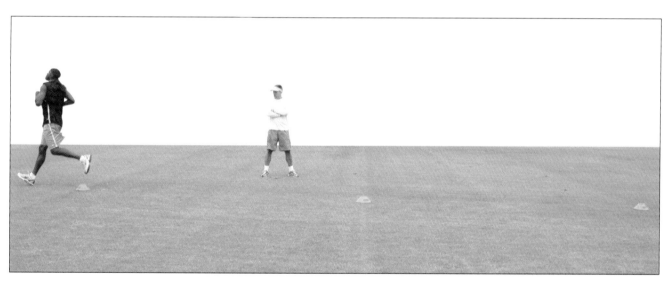

4. Run at the outside cone at full speed. Total distance
of the drill: approximately 15 yards.

71. In-Line Lateral Shuffle

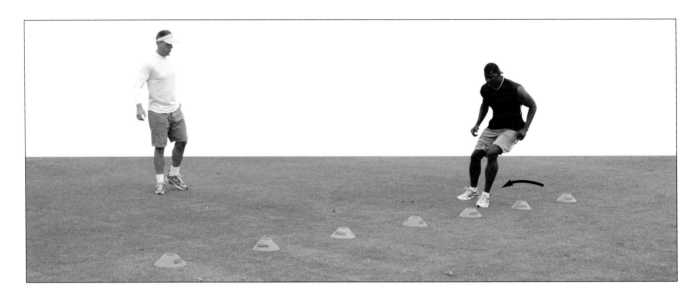

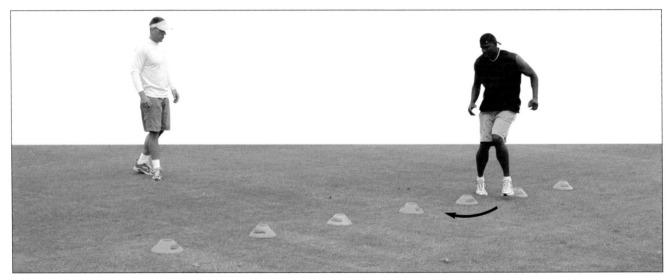

1. Place 8-10 cones approximately 2 feet apart in a straight line. As you begin the drill your feet should be shoulder-width apart. Run around the cones and shuffle your feet to get lateral motion.

QUICK TIPS
- This drill can be completed on sand or on a basketball court as well
- Stay balanced and keep your knees slightly bent as you do the drill

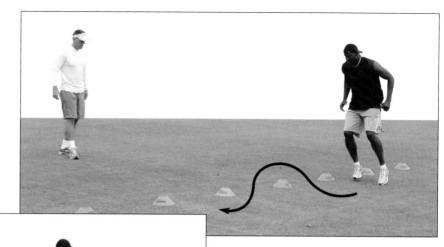

2. As you move through the cones, you should use your arms for balance and speed.

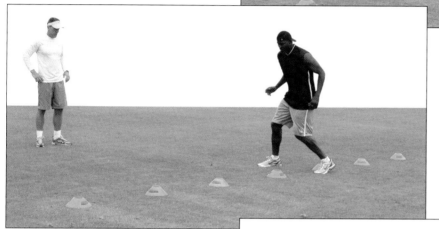

3. It is important that you maintain a good base with your feet. Do not rotate your hips as you move through the cones.

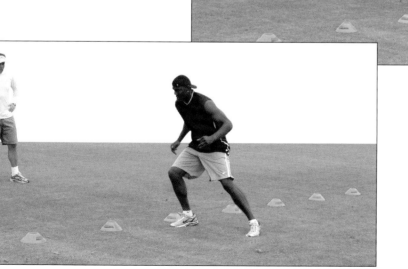

PS

72. In-Line Knee-Ups

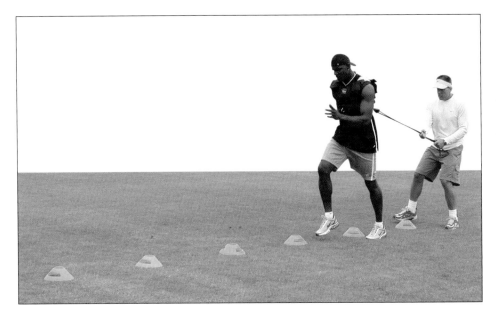

1. Place cones approximately 2 feet apart. Before you begin the drill, place the active leg 8-10 inches behind the support leg. Use a spotter with a harness if you want to add extra resistance.

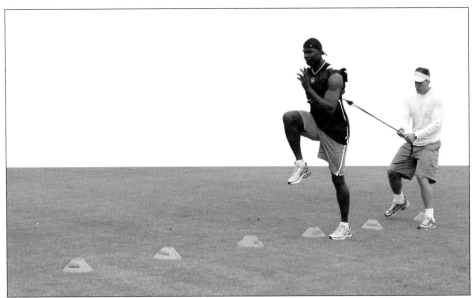

2. As you begin the movement, push off the left leg quickly and lift your working leg (in this case the right) up and over the cones. Step down with your right leg and bring your left one over the next cone. Continue this pattern throughout the drill.

QUICK TIPS
- Work one leg at a time, then go back and repeat the drill focusing on the other leg
- Can be done with or without the vest and cord. Use weighted vest to make the drill more difficult
- Notice the great flexion Keyshawn gets with his active (right) leg

73. Hip Flexion Knee-Ups

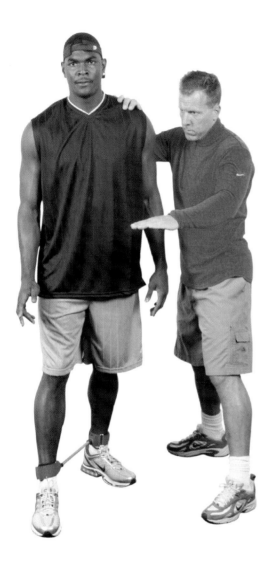
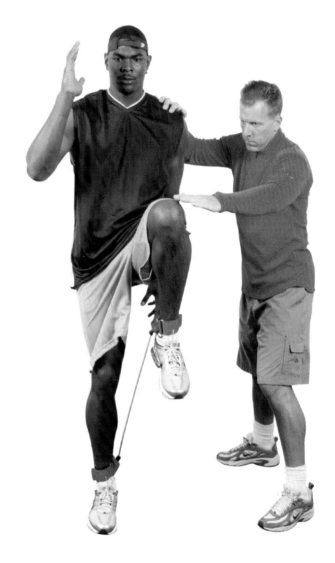

1. Stand with a split stance, holding your hands at waist level. Bring the back leg forward slowly and gently touch the spotter's hand to measure your mark. Return to the start position, ready to begin the movement.

2. Finish: Quickly bring your knee up toward your mark. Once you have touched the mark, return to the starting position. Make sure to work both sides equally.

QUICK TIPS
- Great way to develop hip-flexor strength
- Can be done with or without a bungee cord

PS

74. Medicine Ball Toss-Chest

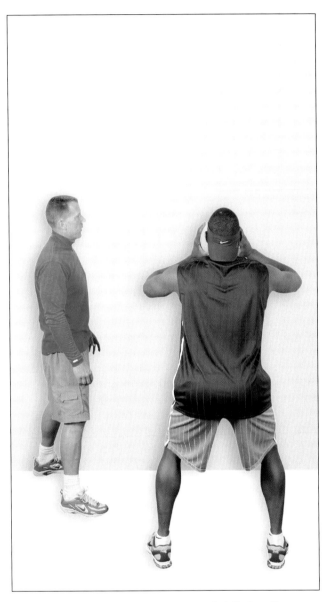 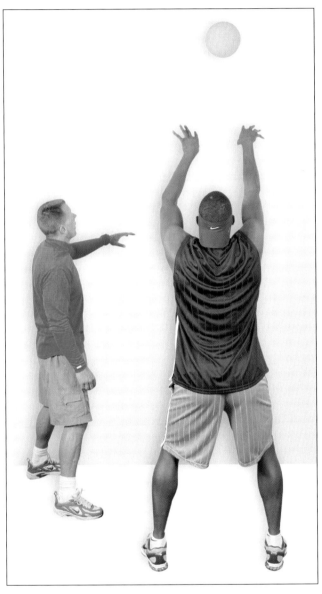

1. Stand in a split or parallel stance, slightly bending your legs in a ready position. Your arms should be flexed. Hold the medicine ball firmly with both hands at chest level.

2. In a quick motion, extend your arms and legs to a split stance, throwing the medicine ball against a wall in an upward plane. Once you release the ball, quickly reposition your hands and feet and be ready to receive the medicine ball from the spotter and repeat the process.

QUICK TIPS
- Good upper body plyometric exercise
- Can throw against a concrete wall for fast repetition, benefiting conditioning
- Can use the split or parallel stance
- Intermediate/Advanced

75. Medicine Ball Toss–Overhead

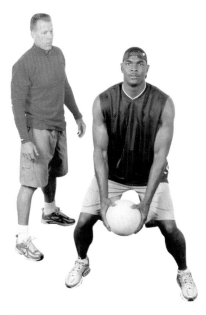

1. Squat with your feet slightly wider than shoulder-width and your thighs parallel to the floor. Your arms are completely extended, holding the medicine ball down below the knees.

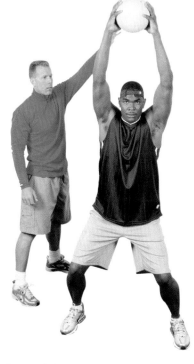

2. In a quick motion, extend your legs, bringing your arms up with great force. Your arms should be flexed until slightly before the release point.

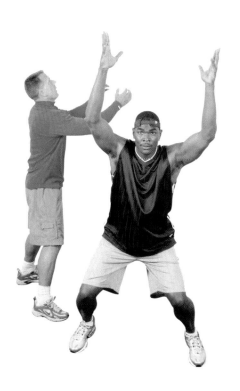

QUICK TIPS
- Can throw against a concrete wall for fast repetition, benefiting conditioning
- Good upper-body plyometric exercise
- Great for upper-body explosiveness
- Intermediate/Advanced

3. Upon releasing the medicine ball, your arms should be straight above your head. You should be up on your toes with a slight backward lean. Your spotter retrieves the medicine ball.

76. Medicine Ball Partner Toss

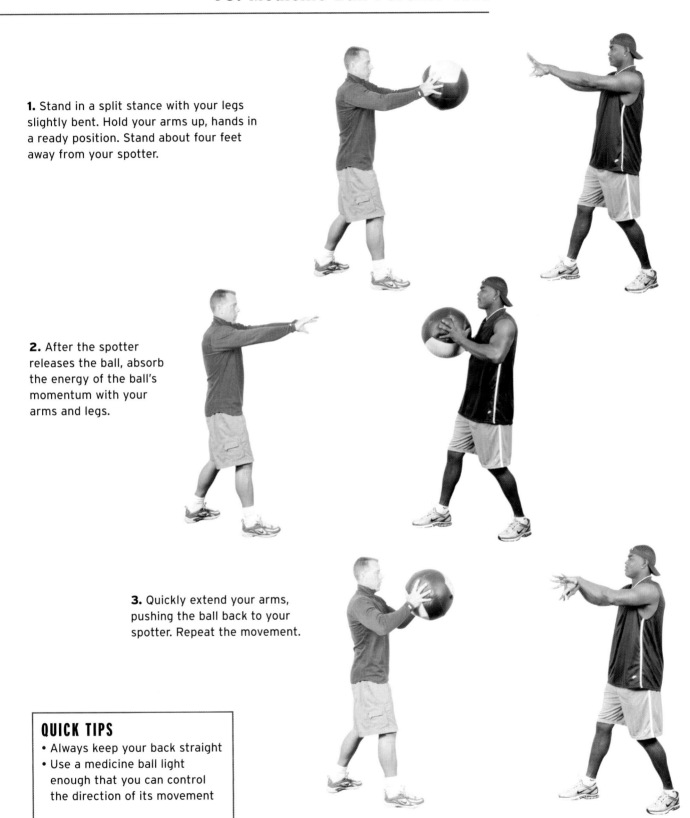

1. Stand in a split stance with your legs slightly bent. Hold your arms up, hands in a ready position. Stand about four feet away from your spotter.

2. After the spotter releases the ball, absorb the energy of the ball's momentum with your arms and legs.

3. Quickly extend your arms, pushing the ball back to your spotter. Repeat the movement.

QUICK TIPS
• Always keep your back straight
• Use a medicine ball light enough that you can control the direction of its movement

77. Squats–Medicine Ball or Plate

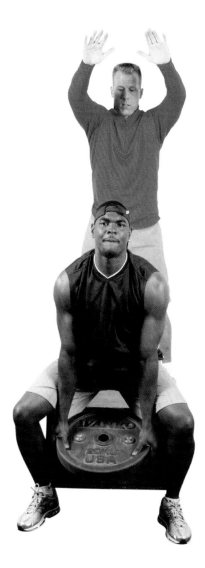 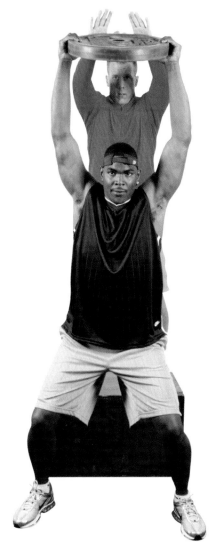

1. The spotter stands directly behind the lifter, with his hands held above the lifter. The lifter should take a shoulder-width stance with thighs parallel to the floor and keep the feet flat on the floor. Hold the medicine ball or plate firmly with both hands in front of you down between the legs. The spotter can stand on a bench or box.

2. Before you begin the exercise, make sure the weight touches the spotter's hands at the highest point. With one quick but controlled motion, stand upright, raising the weight above your head. Once the weight has touched the spotter's hands, return to the starting position.

QUICK TIPS
• Always use a spotter
• Great endurance exercise
• Great total body exercise
• Intermediate/Advanced

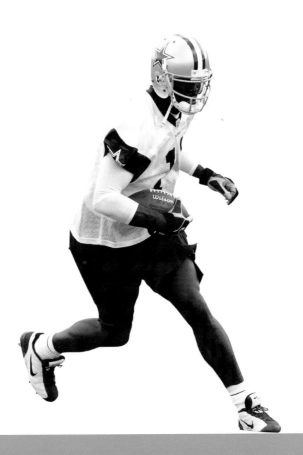

FIELD WORK

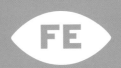

78. Cat and Dog Drill

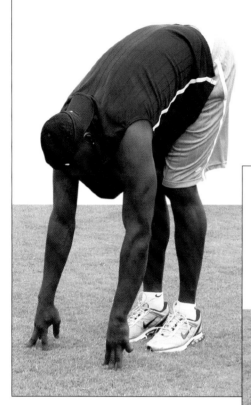

1. Bend at the waist and touch the ground with your hands.

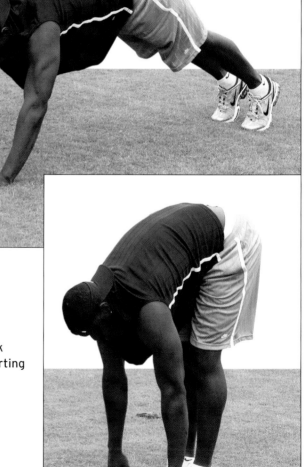

2. Walk your hands forward until you reach a comfortable body extension.

3. Keeping the palms on the ground, walk your feet forward until you reach the starting position.

79. Figure 8's

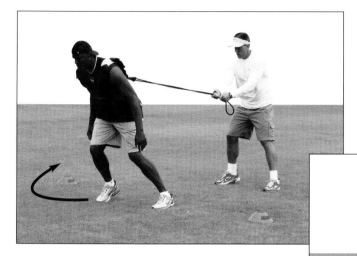

1. Set 2 cones on the ground approximately 3-5 yards apart. Stand between the cones to start shuffling your feet from the outside to the inside. Run in a figure 8 pattern. Repeat in both directions.

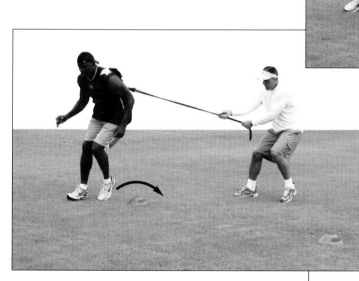

QUICK TIPS
• Can be used with vest or no vest

FE

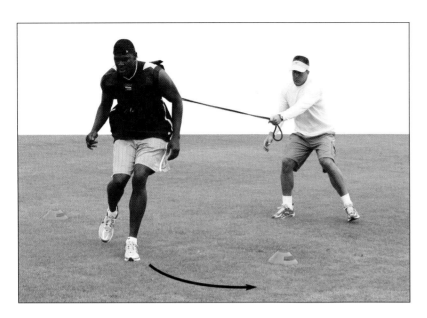

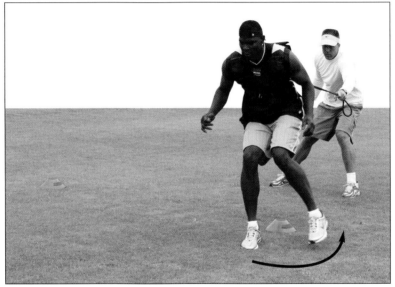

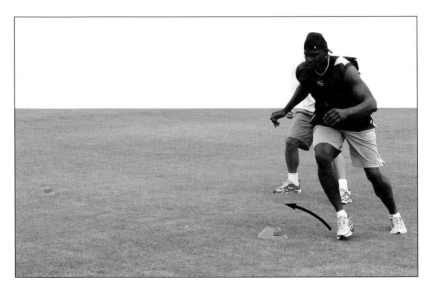

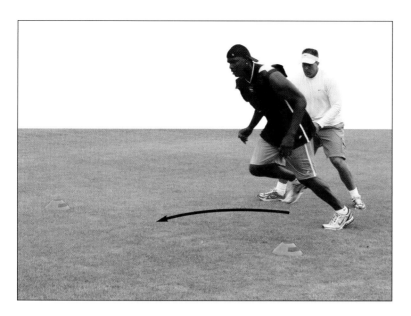

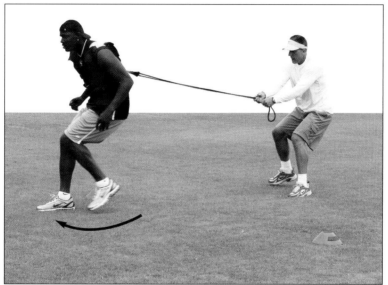

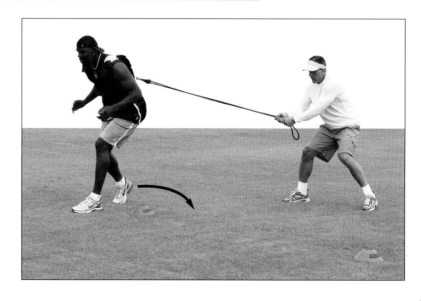

80. Diagonal Shuffle

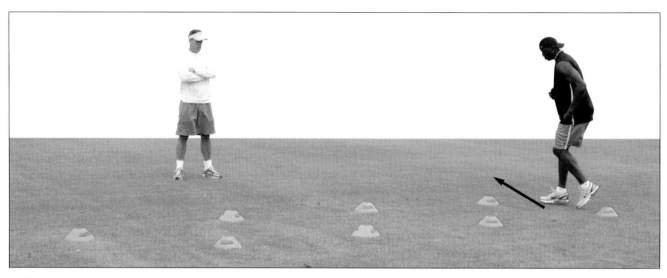

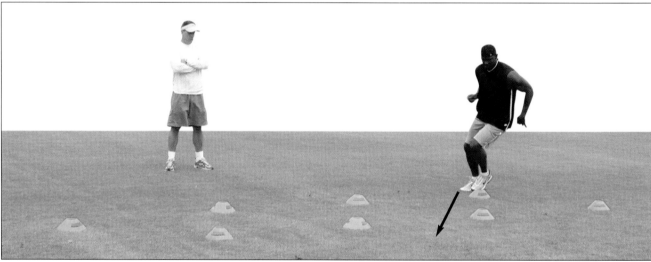

1. Place 8-10 cones in a diagonal pattern. The cones should be staggered and about 3 feet apart. Start running in diagonal cuts as you shuffle through the cones.

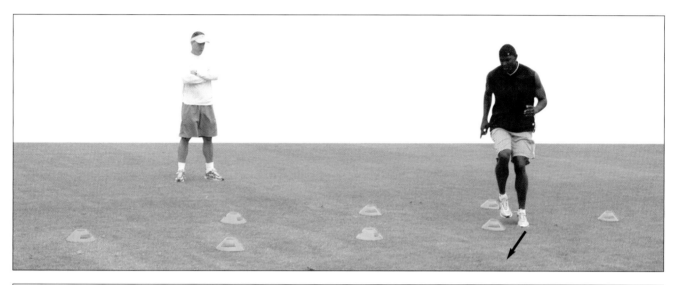

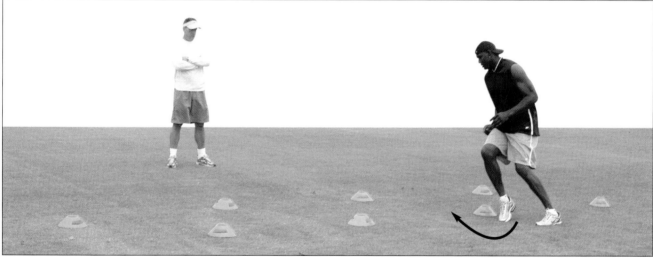

2. As you shuffle through the cones, makes sure you go around the outside of the cones and use your arms for balance and speed.

FE

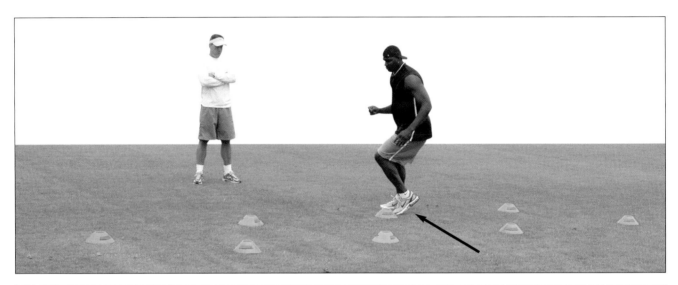

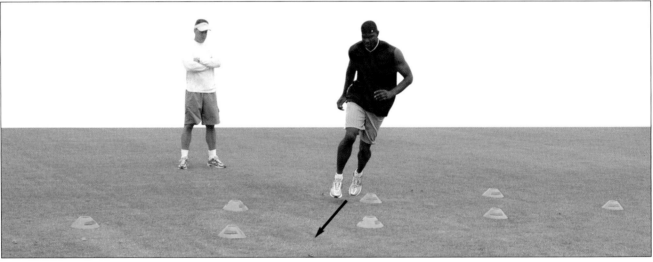

3. Maintain a good base with your feet. Do not rotate your hips as you move through the cones.

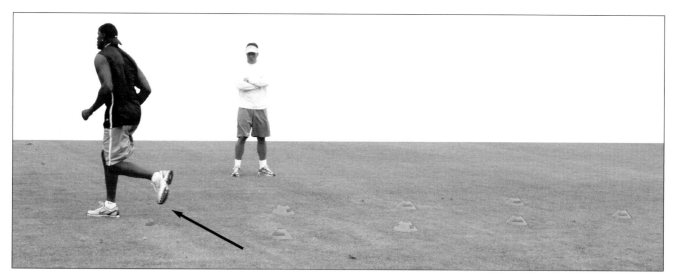

4. Finish the drill powerfully and quickly.

81. V-Jumps

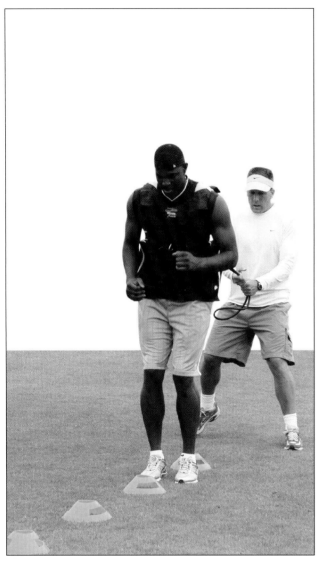

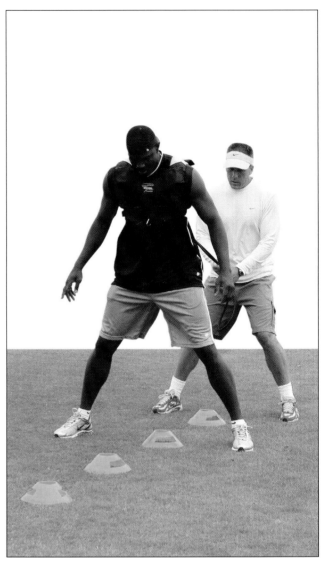

1. Place 8-10 cones approximately 2 feet apart in a straight line. Before you begin, your feet should be about 6-8 inches apart. Your partner holds on to the bungee cord for extra resistance, controlling the resistance according to your level of fitness and agility.

2. As you begin your initial jump, look for your landmark (the next cone). Jump forward and out, landing with your feet straddling the cone. Upon landing, your feet should be wider than shoulder-width.

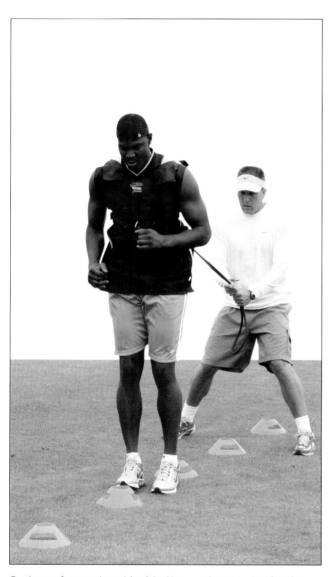

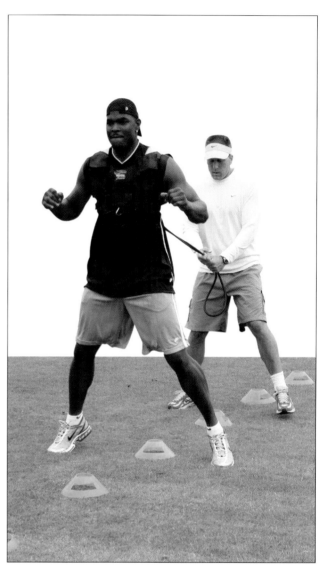

3. Jump forward and inside the next cone. Again visualize your target before you take the jump. Alternate jumping in and out as you jump forward. As you move through the drill, your movements should become quick and explosive.

4. Bend your knees and explode forward on each jump.

FE

82. In-Line Vertical Jumps

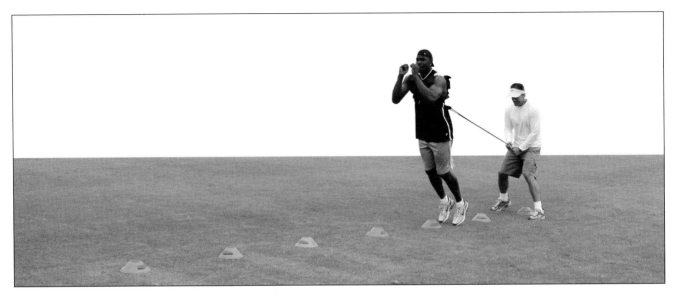

1. Place 8-10 cones approximately 2 feet apart in a straight line. Stand at the first cone, bend your knees, and jump forward.

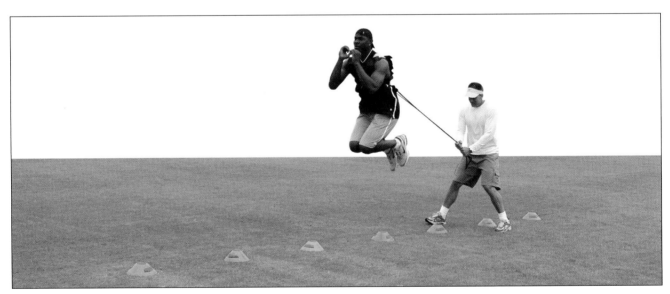

2. As you begin your jump, use your arms to generate even greater momentum and explosion. Land in between each cone.

QUICK TIPS
- This drill can be completed with or without a vest and cord. For extra punch have your trainer or training partner hold the bungee and control the pressure
- Great way to increase your vertical jump

83. Run-Stop

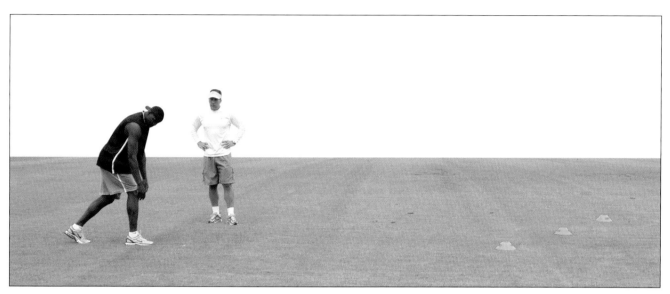

1. Place 3 cones at increasing distances from the starting point (in this case, 5, 7 and 10 yards from the starting point). Position your body so that you can quickly accelerate to the first cone (5 yards).

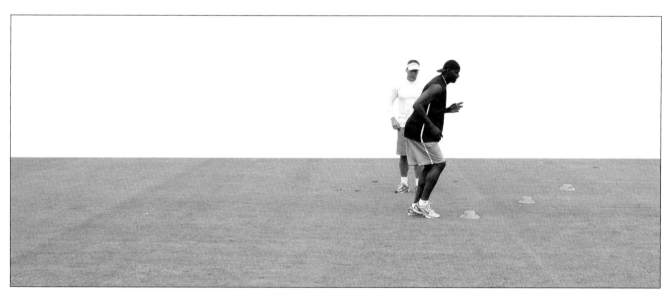

2. As you reach the first cone, rapidly decelerate. Walk back to the starting point. Repeat the process to the cones at 7 and 10 yards. Vary the distance during different workouts so you can develop acceleration for different routes.

FE

84. Key's Catching Drills

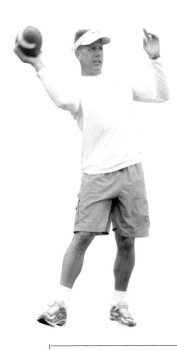

QUICK TIPS
- Always use two hands to catch the ball
- Use an eye patch to make catching more difficult
- Catch the ball with the hands
- Keep the hands soft and suck in the ball, do not try to stop the ball cold when catching it

1. All catches are made at the mid-line of the body.

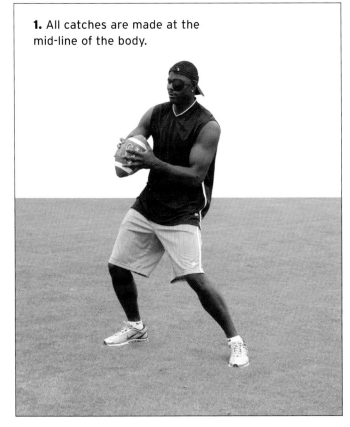

2. All catches are made above the head with fully extended arms.

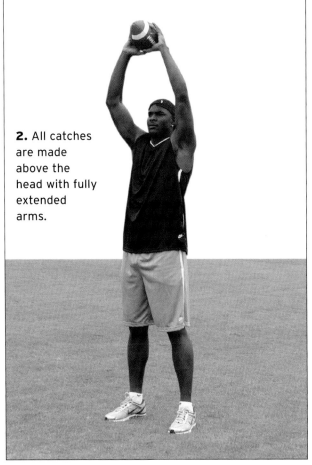

3. All catches are made below the knees with feet slightly wider than shoulder-width apart.

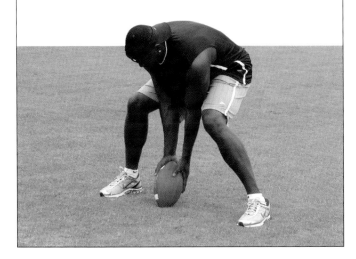

4. Left side catches.

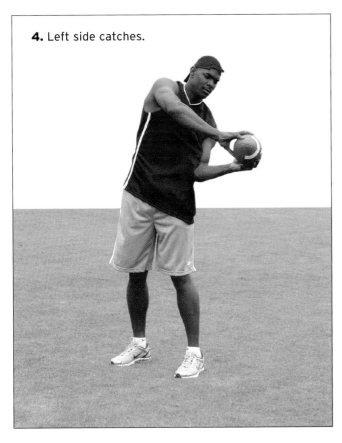

5. Right side catches.

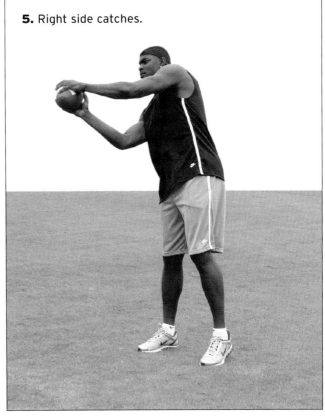

6. Over-the-shoulder right side catches.

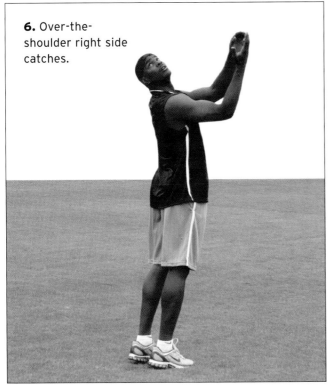

7. Over-the-shoulder left side catches.

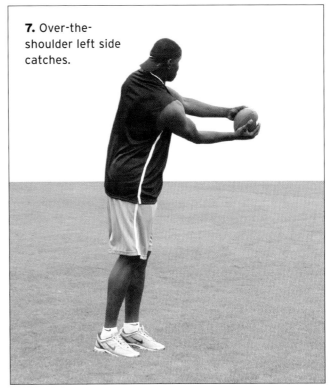

85. Bounce and Catch

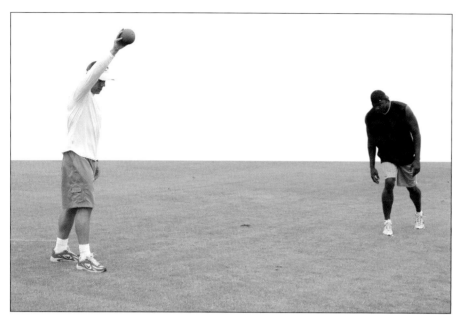

1. Line up 5-6 yards from the ball. Position your feet and body so that you can quickly accelerate when the ball is dropped. The spotter should hold the ball above eye level.

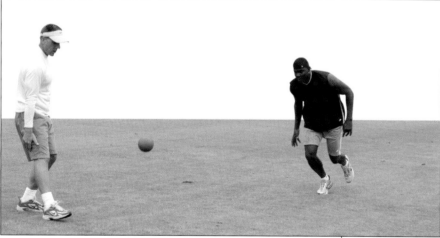

2. As soon as the ball is dropped, accelerate toward the ball, pumping your arms to generate explosive power.

QUICK TIPS
• Keep your eyes on the ball the whole time
• Drive yourself forward to explode off the start
• Spotter may have to throw the ball with some force, depending on the surface (i.e., on hard surfaces you can drop it; on soft surfaces like grass you may have to throw it to get a bounce)

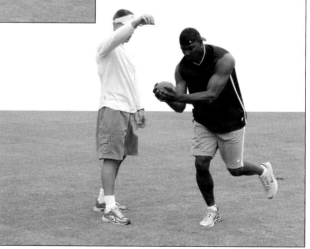

3. After the ball has bounced, reach outward and firmly grab the ball.

PART THREE

PUTTING IT ALL TOGETHER

Most exercise routines have a goal of increasing either power or endurance, but not both. To build power, you reduce the repetitions and increase the weights. To improve endurance, you increase the reps. What makes *our* system unique is that we combine strength, endurance, and power training to make a complete athlete by using different phases of training. That is, for example, for two weeks you may be in a power phase, and then for two weeks you could be in the endurance phase, and then two weeks prior to the season or a competition you combine the two to get optimum performance at that event or be ready for the season.

Whether or not you are an elite athlete like Keyshawn, our system gives you the tools you need to perform in your real world, whatever that world may be. For Keyshawn, it means being able to play for sixty minutes against elite defenders in the NFL, while for someone else it may mean being able to lift boxes at the warehouse, to climb rock walls, or just to be healthy, physically fit, and able to meet life's challenges with confidence. This program will enable you to become functionally strong in the core.

Don't underestimate the importance of organization in your routine. Even if you are a beginner, you need to be organized and have a program so you improve each day. Don't just go out there and do what you feel like doing on a given day. Get a game plan and enough specific guidance so that you know what you need to do to achieve your specific goal. Our system gives you a roadmap; after you start to understand it, you will be able to adapt it to your own changing needs.

One of the major differences between our system and other types of workouts is that ours doesn't divide the training week into specific days for legs or back or chest. We aren't trying to show you how to become a bodybuilder or to sculpt your body to some standard. Rather, our goal is to make you a more fit person or a better athlete, and people use all their body parts in everyday life. So our workouts tax your entire body every session. They are much more demanding! Sure, some days you might do more leg work than others, but overall the workouts are balanced because the tool you use is a single body, not a bunch of parts. In our system, all types of exercises described earlier have been carefully integrated to help you develop the functional power you need.

Additionally, when your workouts concentrate on one specific body part at a time, you don't put your cardio system through its maximum range. What you need to do is to use all your body parts each day to get your system used to supporting your whole body, which will further develop your conditioning.

You need to develop strength and endurance to maintain a weight program, but you also must develop coordination. You may start to realize that your body was not balanced, that, for instance, your left side was weaker than your right side—a realization that comes when you are doing dumbbell bench presses and one side does not respond as well as the other. This learning curve continues as long as you are doing an exercise program.

Some athletes like to start their program by gaining bulk, doing a lot of weightlifting to gain strength, and then add explosiveness by doing the plyometrics. Then they drop the weight routine down a little and add endurance. This sequence is called tapering. You start with the heavier, slower exercises, then as you get near an event, you start to taper the weight training and increase the explosion/endurance workouts. That way, you develop your endurance while still maintaining the functional power you have gained.

A common mistake athletes make, especially at the intermediate level, is to train hard all the way to the day before competition, leaving them nothing to deliver when it counts. They left it all in the gym. That mistake also leads to injuries, because when you push your body too hard and without a proper taper, you overstress your muscular system and it starts to break down. This happens even at the highest levels of competition. You see it a lot in boxing, where a fighter overtrains, gets to the fight flat, and gets hurt in the ring. Proper tapering is a science; while we offer general guidelines, it is up to each individual to understand what works best for him.

Most of your gains will come in the early stage of fitness training, because everything is brand new to your body. Since you are seeing such big results so quickly, it will be tempting to overdo it. You think, "Well, if I got this result with 50 reps, if I do 100 reps I'll get twice the result!" But that is not the case. It is vital that you restrain yourself, introducing your body gradually to the exercises to familiarize your joints, muscles, and tendons with the movements and resistance. Typically, most injuries and gains occur in the early phases of training. Therefore, it is very important to take it slow so you avoid injuries that can set you back tremendously.

Focus

The challenge is to have a program and a series of exercises that are not dull or boring. You must not only get the benefits of the workouts but actually enjoy doing them. This helps you stay focused. If you do exercises that do not challenge you, like too many machine exercises, then your workout will become all work and no play, but when you do things like the plyometric exercises, you are constantly challenging yourself to do them properly. You can't just go through the motions; you have to pay attention to what you're doing and get engaged in the process. These types of exercises not only make the workout seems faster and more entertaining, but they also simulate everyday activities much more closely.

One of the difficulties for people in fitness training is to maintain interest in their program, because as you advance in your workouts, the gains get smaller and smaller. The payoff is less obvious, so people sometimes lose interest or think that the program is not working because they got used to constant, observable improvements and changes in their body. One way to combat workout fatigue is to change your workouts regularly. The human body is a very efficient machine and it adapts quickly to everything. When you do one program with the same exercises for a long time, your body adjusts and, as a consequence, you get less benefit from the same exercises. So you need to change things up. Our workouts are designed to give you maximum flexibility in determining your own course of training. Once you have mastered the basic workout, you are encouraged to experiment by replacing the exercises presented in the workouts with others from the same family. For example, you might remove the box jumps (a plyometric exercise) from your routine and replace them with lateral jumps (also a plyo exercise). Use the icons that mark each exercise category to help you swap similar exercises.

Another thing you can change is the order of the exercises. Even a simple modification like that can send your "machine" into a readjustment period and increase the challenge once again. Although typically you should begin a workout with the harder exercises, by simply changing the order of the exercises you are going to create a new challenge—not only for your body but for your mind as well. The next step beyond that is to change to a different program, like going "back" to the beginner series and adapting it to your new level (by increasing the weight load or repetitions). By doing that you are going to once again disturb your "machine" and challenge it to progress and improve. This actually reenergizes your whole system.

Another variation James and Keyshawn are fond of is, instead of doing all the sets of the first exercise, then moving on to the second, and so on, they take the first three exercises and do one set of each. Then they do one set of each again. They continue doing this until they have completed the first three exercises, then move on to the next group of three and repeat the pattern. This varies your workout and challenges your muscles in a new way.

Off-Season Preparation

Keyshawn likes to use five months of the off-season to get into NFL Shape. During the first month, he and James focus his workouts on high reps of low impact exercises, like the bike and treadmill, which get his body back into the program. They might also target areas that Keyshawn injured, like the lower back or thighs, or an area that bothered him toward the end of the season. Already, they work to emphasize his core strength.

Gradually, Keyshawn phases into another regimen, beginning to execute a number of field drills, first without cleats. To begin building strength, he decreases the number of exercise reps and increases his weights. He also increases the fast-twitch muscle exercises like sprinting, plyometrics, and some of the cone drills to work on his explosive power. After a few weeks, he will add his cleats to the field drills and begin to focus the drills on his specific skills. As it gets toward May, he takes a vacation for a week or two.

Come late May or early June, Keyshawn and James get back into it and combine strength and endurance. The length of each workout is increased and Keyshawn begins the running tests required by each team. Although each position may have slightly different tests, a typical test is like a 300-yard shuttle run in which a player runs from one goal line to the other, back to the starting point, and once more to other goal line for a total of 300 yards. Other typical running tests include "gassers," where a player runs the width of the field (53 yards) up to four times, depending on the team, for a total of 212 yards, or "half-gassers." The purpose of the tests is to make sure the guys trained during the off-season and to establish a fitness benchmark for each athlete. Generally, at this level of professional athletics, the players are in contact with their coaches and the team strength coaches throughout the off-season. Keyshawn has mini-camps in April and May where the players go out for a week and run plays, meet with the coaches, spend time with the quarterback, run routes, etc., so they all usually have a pretty good gauge of their fitness at any time during the year.

Everybody who trains seriously tries to improve from year to year, but at Keyshawn's level, the main goal is to keep from getting hurt. You might think that if Keyshawn squatted 350 pounds last year for two reps, James would push him to get 400 pounds this year, but that's just not possible with athletes in top condition. If you have a Ferrari, you don't try to squeeze another 20 hp from it and risk blowing the engine. All you try to do is maintain top condition.

If you are just starting in on a workout program, your regimen is going to look just a little different from Keyshawn's, but there's no reason that it shouldn't be just as challenging and rewarding! You'll need to follow our beginning workouts to develop the fundamentals, and you'll need a good foundation in strength before you can be explosive and be ready to move to the next level. Typically, the beginning exercises are designed to develop this base. As you get into the intermediate and the advanced levels, the workouts become a little harder, a little more demanding, you'll be doing a few more explosive exercises, and the fieldwork becomes a little more involved. Instead of doing one fieldwork exercise per workout, now you'll be doing two or three. The more strength you develop, the better you can do the drills and that is the goal.

The single greatest benefit of the fieldwork exercises is that they prepare you for any sport you play. Whether you compete in volleyball, football, basketball, or martial arts, you must have explosiveness, lateral movement, quick start-stop ability, core strength, balance, and competence, and the fieldwork develops all of these. These exercises ensure that you are working not only one movement, but are going right, left, forward, backward, and are crossing over and jumping. Fieldwork also gets you outside and makes you feel alive. James does a lot of the lateral drills with his fighters and football players, and he's seen how the fieldwork exercises reveal an athlete's dominant side. If, for example, someone can perform a drill more easily when he goes right, James knows to adjust the workout to develop the other side, thus strengthening the player's all-around performance.

No matter what your skill level, it is very important to become aware of any physical weaknesses and let those weaknesses guide your workout strategy. If you sense an imbalance in your strength, for instance, you can use the isolateral exercises to equalize your power. For instance, if you do bench press isolaterals and you notice that you can rip through all eight reps on your right side but you struggle to get the last two on your left, you can begin to push the left side more deliberately. Alternately, in this instance, you could ease up on the weight, then begin building both sides equally, developing the left side until it is as strong as the right before increasing weights again. In any case, concentrate on being able to perform equally well on both sides and always insure proper form and technique.

If you aren't training for a particular event, you need to take breaks from your routine so you don't burn out. After four to six weeks of training, you need to take an active rest for at least two weeks. Active rest can be any exercise that is unrelated to your normal workout routine but that still keeps your muscles working. Racquetball, tennis, basketball, and biking are all good examples of active rest.

Now here is a secret: When you start back up with your weight training routine after two weeks of active rest, start at a lower level than the one you finished with and build back up. Many people err and injure themselves by restarting their workout program at the same weight and intensity at which they stopped. That is a mistake. After the active rest phase, you need to build back up to your best level, which will happen fairly quickly, but don't just jump back into your maximum performance.

Mental Preparation

The other piece of mental training is discipline, which Keyshawn addressed in Part One of this book. It is important to just reiterate here that three things separate the winners from the talkers: discipline, determination, and a good fitness program. You must have discipline and determination to reach the top. If you don't have them, you must at least get a coach to make you have them. You need to associate yourself with someone you respect, who will be your conscience and get you to do the things you wouldn't do on your own. But that still may not be enough. To reach the top levels, you need to have a burning fire inside of you, and no coach can provide that. Some great coaches will find that fire inside you, where you might not locate it yourself, but it must be present somewhere within you if you expect to become a champion.

The Workouts

As we've said, don't do too much too soon! Start slow, and work your way up into winning form. We recommend that beginners start working out three nonconsecutive days a week, for example, Monday, Wednesday, and Friday. As you get to the intermediate level, you should be at four days a week, say Monday, Tuesday, Thursday, and Friday. The advanced practitioner should move up to five or six days a week. Nobody should do seven days a week!

The beginner and intermediate workouts are each four weeks long and should be followed by a two-week active rest break. The advanced workout is designed to be six weeks long—the two weeks described in the routine below, plus four weeks of a stepped-up intermediate routine—and should also be followed by two weeks of active rest. After the rest interval, proceed to the next fitness level if you feel you have achieved it. During each four- or six-week interval, increase the load (weights) as you see necessary, always keeping in mind the rule of thumb of having enough weight so that you can barely do the last rep.

As mentioned earlier, once you are ready to progress from beginner to intermediate or intermediate to advanced, keep in mind that a weight adjustment may be necessary, and even desired, to acclimate yourself to the new routine. So on your first day at the intermediate level, for instance, if the routine feels like it is too much, try easing up on the weights. Perhaps at the end of the beginner's level you were doing lateral raises with 30 pounds on each arm, but the intermediate routine requires a few more reps from you, and the extra requirements are getting to be too much. It may be the time to lower the load for the exercises, even if only temporarily, so that your body can adjust to the new demands.

If you are an advanced practitioner, or a beginner or intermediate who wants to stay at your present workout level for another four weeks before advancing, remember to modify your routine. The workouts at all levels are designed with this flexibility in mind. As noted previously, if you need to alter your workout to fight workout fatigue, you can modify your routine in three distinct ways. First, you can always alter the sequence of the specified exercises. Second, you can increase the difficulty of a given exercise. For example, the free-weights exercise Front Raises can be executed with the barbell, dumbbells, plates, or isolaterally. If you are a beginner, start with the easiest options (dumbbells, then isolaterally with dumbbells). As you get more advanced, proceed to the more difficult options (plates and barbell). Finally, you can use the icons to substitute one exercise for another in the same family. In the intermediate workout, for instance, Week 1 Day 3 calls for plyometrics. You could easily replace one or several of the plyometric exercises with others from the plyometrics category in Part Two to design a new workout! The Box Jumps (59) could be replaced with Lateral Jumps (61). You could even turbocharge into a Power Series exercise, such as the In-Line Knee-Ups (72). The icons will also help advanced practitioners, who are directed after the first two weeks to go back and use the intermediate four-week program, adding an exercise of the same group to each day's routine.

To get the maximum benefits of our program, you should end each workout with the cardiovascular conditioning exercises that are specified. However, there are times when this will not be possible, and in those cases it is okay to do the cardio part at a different time. In either case, don't forget to warm up and stretch!

Each line in the workouts below represents a complete exercise. For example, in the line

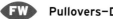 **Pullovers—Dumbbell (30):** 10; 10; 10

the first item is the title (Pullovers—Dumbbell), and the number in parenthesies (in this case, 30) refers to the exercise number in Part Two. If a title is not followed by a number, we assume you need no explanation of the exercise. Such is the case, for example, with pull-ups. The numbers following the colon are the repetitions for each set. The pullovers exercise above specifies 3 sets of 10 repetitions, meaning that you would do 10 reps of the exercise for the first set, rest for a pre-established period, then do 2 more sets of 10 reps each, followed by proper rest to complete that exercise before proceeding to the next exercise of that day's workout. The icon on each line will help you exchange exercises when you are ready to modify your workout.

Proper rest intervals depend on each individual. For beginners, we recommend between one and two minutes of rest between sets and at least two minutes between exercises. If after two minutes you don't feel ready to go on, you should wait and collect yourself before proceeding. Conversely, if after 30 seconds you feel ready to rock, then go ahead. It is important that you learn to adjust the rest time to best fit your body and fitness level. Another way to set rest intervals, of course, is to use a heartbeat monitor and set a desired heartbeat level of rest. In other words, let's say you set 100 hbpm (heartbeats per minute) as your rest level, then you would do the exercise and, upon finishing it, rest until your heartbeat gets down to that level. This is more advanced, but it is a very effective method of pushing your limits, especially in plyometric exercises and interval training.

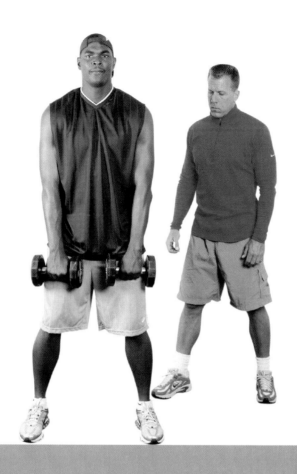

Beginner Workout–3 days/week

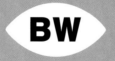

At the end of the four weeks of Beginner Workout, take two weeks of active rest doing an activity that you prefer—like biking, running, swimming, or playing tennis—before you advance to the intermediate workout. If you feel you are not ready to proceed to the intermediate workout routine yet, repeat the four weeks of the beginner workout but replace at least one exercise in each workout day with another one of the same family, or simply alter the exercise order to challenge your system a little more.

Day 1

Warm-Up

CC   **Jump Rope (13):** 45 seconds; 45 seconds; 45 seconds

or

FW   **Lunges–Body Weight (27):** 10 reps per side; 10 reps per side; 10 reps per side

Stretch

KSR   **Keyshawn Stretch Routine**

Mental Training

Believe in yourself: Think back to a time when your perseverance led to success. Remember how it felt to believe in yourself and achieve your goal.

Strength Training–Chest and Back

FW   **Curls–Towel (43):** 12; 12; 12; 10; 10; 10

or

FW   **Pullovers–Dumbbell (30):** 10; 10; 10

PL   **Push-Ups–Plyometric (64):** 10-15; 10-15; 10-15

FW   **Bench Press–Barbell (21):** 10; 10; 10

Strength Training–Legs

FW   **Squats–Body Weight (37):** 15-20; 15-20; 15-20

Abdominals

AB   **High Crunches (1):** 15-20; 15-20; 15-20

Cardiovascular Conditioning

CC   **Steady Run or Jog (15b):** 10-12 minutes

PS   **In-Line Lateral Shuffle (71):** 20 seconds, rest 1:30; 20 seconds, rest 1:30; 20 seconds, rest 1:30

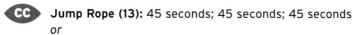
Warm-Up

CC Jump Rope (13): 45 seconds; 45 seconds; 45 seconds
or
PL Step-Ups (60): 8-10 per leg; 8-10 per leg; 8-10 per leg

Stretch

KSR Keyshawn Stretch Routine

Mental Training

Put worry where it belongs: Remember a situation in which you worried and reflect on whether the worry affected the situation's outcome.

Strength Training–Shoulders

FW Lateral Raise–Dumbbell (26): 10; 10; 10
or
FW Front Raise–Dumbbell (23): 10; 10; 10

FW Shoulder Shrugs–Dumbbell (36): 10; 10; 10

FW Military Press–Dumbbell (29): 10; 10; 10

Strength Training–Plyometrics

PL Box Jumps–Small Box (59a): 8; 8; 8

FE V-Jumps (81): 10-16; 10-16; 10-16

Cardiovascular Conditioning

CC Steady Run or Jog (15b): 10-12 minutes

Warm-Up

CC **Jump Rope (13):** 45 seconds; 45 seconds; 45 seconds
or
FW **Lunges–Body Weight (27):** 10 reps per side; 10 reps per side; 10 reps per side

Stretch

KSR **Keyshawn Stretch Routine**

Mental Training

Identify your strengths: Think of something you have done well and identify what enables you to do it well. What does it feel like to be engaged in a task that you do well?

Strength Training–Chest/Back/Legs

FW **Pullovers–Dumbbell (30):** 10; 10; 10

PL **Push-Ups–Plyometric (64):** 10-15; 10-15; 10-15

FW **Bench Press–Barbell (21):** 10; 10; 10

FW **High Pull–Dumbbell (24):** 10; 10; 10

PS **Squats–Medicine Ball or Plate (77):** 15-20; 15-20; 15-20

Abdominals

AB **High Crunches (1):** 15-20; 15-20; 15-20

Cardiovascular Conditioning

CC **Steady Run or Jog (15b):** 12 minutes

PS **In-Line Lateral Shuffle (71):** 20 seconds; 20 seconds; 20 seconds

Warm-Up

CC **Steady Run or Jog (15b):** 5 minutes

FE **Key's Catching Drills (84):** Choose 2 drills, 30 catches each way

Stretch

KSR Keyshawn Stretch Routine

Mental Training

Create success: Visualize achieving a specific goal or winning an upcoming competition.

Strength Training–Plyometrics

PS **3-Cone Drill (67):** 3 reps, 60-second rest between reps

PL **Medicine Ball Ground Work–One Hand (62):** 15 seconds; 15 seconds; 15 seconds

PS **Medicine Ball Partner Toss (76):** 8-12; 8-12; 8-12

FW **Rice Grabs (33):** 30 seconds; 30 seconds; 30 seconds

Abdominals

AB **Roll-Ups (4):** 15-20; 15-20; 15-20

Cardiovascular Conditioning

CC **Sprints (16):** 8-10 sprints, 100 yards each. Walk back to starting point.

Day 2

Warm-Up

FW **Rice Grabs (33):** 30 seconds; 30 seconds; 30 seconds

PS **4-Cone Drill (68):** 5 sets, 60-second rest between sets

Stretch

KSR Keyshawn Stretch Routine

Mental Training

Seek inspiration: Pick one of the quotes in this book and reflect on how it pertains to a specific circumstance in your life.

Strength Training—Shoulders and Legs

FW **Lateral Raise—Dumbbell (26):** 10; 10; 10

FW **Front Raise—Dumbbell (23):** 10; 10; 10

FW **Shoulder Shrugs—Dumbbell (36):** 10; 10; 10

FW **Military Press—Dumbbell (29):** 10; 10; 10; 10

FW **Upright Row—Barbell (41):** 10; 10; 10

FW **Squats—Dumbbell (38):** 10; 10; 10; 10

Abdominals

AB **Roll-Ups (4):** 15-20; 15-20; 15-20

Cardiovascular Conditioning

CC **Steady Run or Jog (15b):** 15-18 minutes

Warm-Up

FW **Rice Grabs (33):** 30 seconds; 30 seconds; 30 seconds

FW **Lunges—Body Weight (27):** 10 reps per side; 10 reps per side; 10 reps per side

Stretch

KSR **Keyshawn Stretch Routine**

Mental Training

Don't settle for less than you can be: Identify one thing in your life that you can do better. Identify two ways to improve your work in that area and put them into play.

Strength Training—Chest and Back

FW **Pullovers—Towel (31):** 12; 12; 12

FW **Bench Press—Dumbbell (22):** 10; 10; 10; 10

FW **High Pull—Dumbbell (24):** 8; 8; 8

FW **Incline Press—Dumbbell (25):** 10; 10; 10

FW **Pull-Ups:** 4-8; 4-8; 4-8

Abdominals

AB **High Crunches (1):** 15-20; 15-20; 15-20

AB **Roll-Ups (4):** 15-20; 15-20; 15-20

Cardiovascular Conditioning

CC **Steady Run or Jog (15b):** 15-18 minutes

PS **3-Cone Drill (67):** 4 reps, 60-second rest between reps

Day 1

Warm-Up

FW **Rice Grabs (33):** 30 seconds; 30 seconds; 30 seconds

PS **3-Way Warm-Up (66):** 4 sets, 60-second rest between each set

Stretch

KSR **Keyshawn Stretch Routine**

Mental Training

Don't let others tell you what you can or can't do.

Strength Training–Shoulders and Legs

FW **Front Raise–Dumbbell (23):** 10; 10; 10

FW **Lateral Raise–Dumbbell (26):** 10; 10; 10

FW **Military Press–Dumbbell (29):** 10; 10; 8; 8

FW **Upright Row–Plate (41):** 10; 10; 10

FW **Lunges–Body Weight (27):** 10 reps per side; 10 reps per side; 10 reps per side

FW **Straight-Leg Dead Lifts–Dumbbell (40):** 10; 10; 10

Cardiovascular Conditioning

CC **Sprints (16):** 8-10 sprints, 100 yards each. Walk back to starting point.

Warm-Up

CC **Steady Run or Jog (15b):** 5 minutes

FE **Key's Catching Drills (84):** Choose 2 drills, 30 catches each way

Stretch

KSR **Keyshawn Stretch Routine**

Mental Training

Demand a lot from yourself: Beginning with one exercise in today's workout, push yourself beyond your comfort zone.

Strength Training–Plyometrics

PS **3-Cone Drill (67):** 3 reps, 60-second rest between reps

PS **Medicine Ball Partner Toss (76):** 10-15; 10-15; 10-15

PL **Lateral Jumps–Long Way (61):** 12-16; 12-16; 12-16

CC **Jump Rope (13):** 45 seconds; 45 seconds; 45 seconds

PL **Medicine Ball Ground Work–One Hand (62):** 20 seconds; 20 seconds; 20 seconds

Abdominals

AB **Roll-Ups (4):** 12-15; 12-15; 12-15

Cardiovascular Conditioning

CC **Steady Run or Jog (15b):** 15-18 minutes

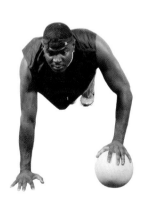
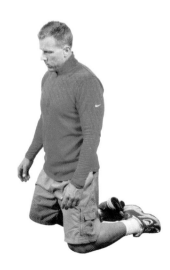

Warm-Up

CC **Jump Rope (13):** 45 seconds; 45 seconds; 45 seconds
or
FW **Lunges–Body Weight (27):** 10 reps per side; 10 reps per side; 10 reps per side

Stretch

KSR **Keyshawn Stretch Routine**

Mental Training

Identify your dreams: Pick a current project or short-term objective.
Visualize what you want to happen and imagine yourself achieving your goal.

Strength Training–Chest/Back/Legs

FW **Row–Dumbbell (34):** 10; 10; 10
or
FW **Pullovers–Towel (31):** 12; 12; 12

PL **Push-Ups–Plyometric (64):** 10-15; 10-15; 10-15

FW **Bench Press–Barbell (21):** 10; 10; 10

PS **Squats–Medicine Ball or Plate (77):** 15-20; 15-20; 15-20

Abdominals

AB **High Crunches (1):** 15-20; 15-20; 15-20

Cardiovascular Conditioning

CC **Steady Run or Jog (15b):** 15-20 minutes

Warm-Up

FW **Rice Grabs (33):** 30 seconds; 30 seconds; 30 seconds

FW **Lunges–Body Weight (27):** 10 reps per side; 10 reps per side; 10 reps per side

Stretch

KSR **Keyshawn Stretch Routine**

Mental Training

Learn from your setbacks: Think of a situation that went wrong. What have you changed since that occurred? What were the lessons learned from it? How are you planning to keep that mistake from happening again?

Strength Training–Chest and Back

FW **Pullovers–Dumbbell (30):** 10; 10; 10

FW **Incline Press–Dumbbell (25):** 10; 10; 10

FW **High Pull–Dumbbell (24):** 8; 8; 8

FW **Bench Press–Dumbbell (22):** 10; 10; 10; 10

FW **Pull-Ups:** 4-8; 4-8; 4-8

Abdominals

AB **High Crunches (1):** 15-20; 15-20; 15-20

AB **Roll-Ups (4):** 15-20; 15-20; 15-20

Cardiovascular Conditioning

CC **Steady Run or Jog (15b):** 15-18 minutes

PS **In-Line Lateral Shuffle (71):** 20 seconds; 20 seconds; 20 seconds, 60-second rest between reps

BW

Day 2

Warm-Up

CC **Run in Place (14)** *or* **Steady Run or Jog (15b):** 5 minutes

Stretch

KSR Keyshawn Stretch Routine

Mental Training

Develop a winning attitude: Identify one area of improvement in your workouts. Apply the confidence you gain from realizing your progress to any areas in the workout that are especially challenging.

Strength Training—Grip and Shoulders

PL **Medicine Ball Ground Work—One Hand (62):** 12-15 reps; 12-15 reps; 12-15 reps

FW **Rice Grabs (33):** 30 seconds; 30 seconds; 30 seconds

PS **Medicine Ball Partner Toss (76):** 8-12; 8-12; 8-12

FW **Lateral Raise—Dumbbell (26):** 10; 10; 10

FW **Upright Row—Barbell (41):** 10; 10; 10

FW **Shoulder Shrugs—Dumbbell (36):** 10; 10; 10

FW **Military Press—Dumbbell (29):** 10; 10; 8; 8

Abdominals

AB **Good Mornings (2):** 12; 12; 12

Cardiovascular Conditioning

CC **Sprints (16):** 8-10 sprints, 100 yards each. Walk back to starting point.

Warm-Up

FW **Rice Grabs (33):** 30 seconds; 30 seconds; 30 seconds

FW **Lunges–Body Weight (27):** 10 reps per side; 10 reps per side; 10 reps per side

Stretch

KSR **Keyshawn Stretch Routine**

Mental Training

Never forget who you are: What did friends from your youth say your best characteristic was? Do you still have that quality? Are you still in touch with your old friends? Call an old friend today!

Strength Training–Chest/Back/Legs

PL **Push-Ups–Plyometric (64):** 12-15; 12-15; 12-15

FW **Row–Dumbbell (34):** 10; 10; 10

FW **Bench Press–Barbell (21):** 10; 10; 10

FW **Pullovers–Towel (31):** 12; 12; 12

FW **Squats–Dumbbell (38):** 10; 10; 10; 10

PL **Step-Ups (60):** 10-12 per leg; 10-12 per leg; 10-12 per leg

Cardiovascular Conditioning

CC **Steady Run or Jog (15b):** 15-18 minutes

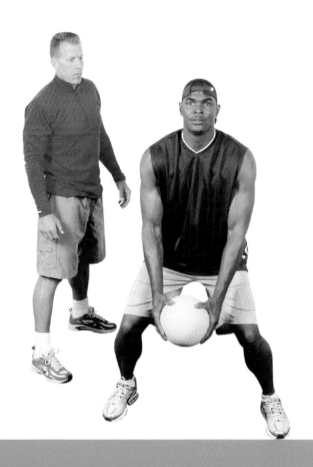

Intermediate Workout–4 days/week

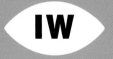

IW

At the end of the four-week routine described here, take two weeks of active rest doing an activity that you enjoy—like bicycling, running, swimming, or playing tennis—before you move on to the advanced workout. If you feel you are not ready to proceed to the advanced workout routine yet, repeat the four weeks in the intermediate workout and replace at least one exercise in each workout day with another one of the same family, or simply alter the exercise order to challenge your system a little more.

Day 1

Warm-Up

FE **Key's Catching Drills (84):** Choose 4 drills, 20 catches each way

AB **Good Mornings (2):** 10; 10; 10

CC **Jump Rope (13):** 60 seconds; 60 seconds; 60 seconds

Stretch

KSR **Keyshawn Stretch Routine**

Mental Training

Believe in yourself: Identify the toughest challenge in today's workout. Visualize yourself accomplishing the reps with ease.

Strength Training—Chest/Back/Legs

FW **Straight-Leg Dead Lifts—Dumbbell (40):** 10; 10; 10

FW **Squats—Dumbbell (38):** 10; 10; 10; 10

ME **Leg Extension (56):** 12; 12; 12

PL **Box Jumps—Big Box (59b):** 8-10; 8-10; 8-10

ISO **Bench Press—Isolateral (45):** 10; 8; 8; 6; 6

FW **Pullovers—Dumbbell (30):** 8; 8; 8; 8

ISO **Incline Press—Isolateral (47):** 8; 8; 8; 8

FW **Pull-Ups:** 6-8; 6-8; 6-8

Abdominals

AB **High Crunches (1):** 20; 20; 20

Cardiovascular Conditioning

CC **Steady Run or Jog (15b):** 5-8 minutes

CC **Sprints (16):** 4-6 sprints, 200 yards each. Walk back to starting point.

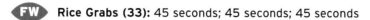

Warm-Up

FW **Rice Grabs (33):** 45 seconds; 45 seconds; 45 seconds

PL **Step-Ups (60):** 25 seconds; 25 seconds; 25 seconds; 25 seconds

Stretch

KSR **Keyshawn Stretch Routine**

Mental Training

Put worry where it belongs: Identify something that concerns you. Are you worried about it? Identify one action you could take to improve the situation and resolve to put it into play after the workout.

Strength Training–Shoulders

ISO **Front Raise–Isolateral (46):** 10; 10; 10; 10

FW **Lateral Raise–Dumbbell (26):** 10; 10; 10; 10

ISO **Military Press–Isolateral (49):** 8; 8; 6; 6

FW **High Pull–Dumbbell (24):** 6; 6; 6; 6

FW **Shoulder Shrugs–Dumbbell (36):** 10; 10; 10; 10

FW **Power Clean–Barbell (44):** 4; 4; 4; 4

Abdominals

AB **V-Ups (5):** 12-15; 12-15; 12-15; 12-15

Cardiovascular Conditioning

CC **Steady Run or Jog (15b):** 5-8 minutes

CC **Sprints (16):** 4-6 sprints, 200 yards each. Walk back to starting point.

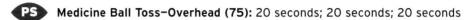

Warm-Up

PS   **Medicine Ball Toss—Overhead (75):** 20 seconds; 20 seconds; 20 seconds

CC   **Jump Rope (13):** 60 seconds; 60 seconds; 60 seconds

Stretch

KSR   **Keyshawn Stretch Routine**

Mental Training

Identify your strengths: Think of a task you accomplish easily. Reflect on whether you could apply the characteristic that makes you effective with this task to other parts of your life.

Strength Training—Plyometrics

PS   **Medicine Ball Toss—Overhead (75):** 20 seconds; 20 seconds; 20 seconds

PL   **Lateral Jumps—Long Way (61):** 20 seconds; 20 seconds; 20 seconds; 20 seconds

FW   **Lunges—Body Weight (27):** 15-20 yards; 15-20 yards; 15-20 yards; 15-20 yards

PL   **Box Jumps—Big Box (59b):** 8-10; 8-10; 8-10

PS   **Medicine Ball Partner Toss (76):** 30 seconds; 30 seconds; 30 seconds

FE   **V-Jumps (81):** 20 seconds; 20 seconds; 20 seconds; 20 seconds

Abdominals

AB   **Bent Leg Crunch with Twist (6):** 12-15; 12-15; 12-15

AB   **Decline Bench Crunch with Medicine Ball (7):** 25 seconds; 25 seconds; 25 seconds, 60-second rest between each set

Cardiovascular Conditioning

CC   **Treadmill Workout, Protocol A or B (20)**

Warm-Up

FW **Pullovers—Towel (31):** 12; 12; 12

AB **Good Mornings (2):** 10; 10; 10

Mental Training

Create incremental success: Choose an exercise from today's workout. Identify your comfort zone with that exercise and plan to go just a little beyond it today. Don't stretch too far. Create the opportunity to experience incremental success.

Stretch

KSR **Keyshawn Stretch Routine**

Strength Training—Chest/Back/Legs

FW **Straight-Leg Dead Lifts—Barbell (39):** 10; 10; 10

PL **Bench Squat with One Leg—Body Weight (65):** 10; 10; 10

FW **Squats—Barbell (37):** 10; 10; 8; 8

PL **Box Jumps—Small or Big (59):** 10-14; 10-14; 10-14

ISO **Bench Press—Isolateral (45):** 10; 8; 6; 6

FW **Row—Dumbbell (34):** 8; 8; 8; 8

ISO **Incline Press—Isolateral (47):** 8; 8; 6; 6

FW **Pull-Ups:** 6-8; 6-8; 6-8

Abdominals

AB **V-Ups (5):** 10-12; 10-12; 10-12; 10-12

Cardiovascular Conditioning

CC **Soft Sand or Grass Run (15a):** 20-30 minutes
or
CC **Treadmill Workout, Protocol A (20)**

IW

Day 1

Warm-Up

FW **Rice Grabs (33):** 45 seconds; 45 seconds; 45 seconds; 45 seconds

PL **Step-Ups (60):** 25 seconds; 25 seconds; 25 seconds; 25 seconds

Mental Training

Seek inspiration: Choose a quote from this book or elsewhere and identify why you like it. In what ways is it pertinent to your present or your past?

Stretch

KSR **Keyshawn Stretch Routine**

Strength Training—Shoulders

ISO **Front Raise—Isolateral (46):** 10; 10; 10; 10

FW **Lateral Raise—Dumbbell (26):** 10; 10; 10; 10

FW **Shoulder Shrugs—Barbell (35):** 10; 10; 10; 10

ISO **Military Press—Isolateral (49):** 8; 6; 6; 6

FW **High Pull—Dumbbell (24):** 6; 6; 6; 6

FW **Power Clean—Barbell (44):** 5; 5; 5; 5

Abdominals

AB **Roll-Ups (4):** 15-20; 15-20; 15-20; 15-20

AB **V-Ups (5):** 10-12; 10-12; 10-12

Cardiovascular Conditioning

CC **Steady Run or Jog (15b):** 5-8 minutes

CC **Sprints (16):** 4-6 sprints, 200 yards each. Walk back to starting point.

Warm-Up

PL **Medicine Ball Ground Work–One Hand (62):** 20 seconds; 20 seconds; 20 seconds

FW **Lunges–Dumbbell (28):** 20 reps per side; 20 reps per side; 20 reps per side

CC **Jump Rope (13):** 60 seconds; 60 seconds; 60 seconds

Mental Training

Don't settle for less than you can be: Identify the most challenging exercise from today's workout. Pinpoint your comfort zone with that exercise and push yourself a little beyond it today.

Stretch

KSR **Keyshawn Stretch Routine**

Strength Training–Chest/Back/Legs

PS **Squats–Medicine Ball or Plate (77):** 15; 15; 15; 15

ME **Leg Extension (56):** 12; 12; 12

FW **Squats–Barbell (37):** 8; 8; 8; 8

ME **Leg Flexion (57):** 12; 12; 12

PL **Box Jumps–Big Box (59b):** 8-10; 8-10; 8-10

FW **Bench Press–Dumbbell (22):** 8; 8; 6; 6; 6

FW **Pullovers–Dumbbell (30):** 8; 8; 8; 8

ISO **Incline Press–Isolateral (47):** 8; 8; 8; 8

FW **Pull-Ups:** 6-8; 6-8; 6-8

Abdominals

AB **High Crunches (1):** 20; 20; 20; 20

Cardiovascular Conditioning

CC **Steady Run or Jog (15b):** 5-8 minutes

CC **Sprints (16):** 4-6 sprints, 200 yards each. Walk back to starting point.

IW

Day 3

Warm-Up

FW Lunges–Body Weight (27)

CC Jump Rope (13): 60 seconds; 60 seconds; 60 seconds

Stretch

KSR Keyshawn Stretch Routine

Mental Training

Demand a lot from yourself: Identify the least challenging exercise from today's workout. Push yourself to do more with that exercise than you have been doing.

Strength Training–Plyometrics

PL Medicine Ball Ground Work–One Hand (62): 20 seconds; 20 seconds; 20 seconds

PL Lateral Jumps–Long Way (61): 20 seconds; 20 seconds; 20 seconds; 20 seconds

FW Squats–Dumbbell (38): 10; 10; 8; 8

PL Box Jumps–Big Box (59b): 8-10; 8-10; 8-10

PS Medicine Ball Partner Toss (76): 30 seconds; 30 seconds; 30 seconds; 30 seconds

FE V-Jumps (81): 20 seconds; 20 seconds; 20 seconds; 20 seconds

Abdominals

AB Medicine Ball Plyometric Oblique Toss (10): 10-12; 10-12; 10-12

AB V-Ups (5): 25; 25; 25

Cardiovascular Conditioning

CC Sprints (16): 4-6 sprints, 200 yards each. Walk back to starting point.

Warm-Up

AB V-Ups (5): 10-12; 10-12; 10-12

FW Rice Grabs (33): 40 seconds; 40 seconds; 40 seconds

Stretch

KSR Keyshawn Stretch Routine

Mental Training

Learn from your setbacks: Bring to mind how you felt the last time you failed at something. Remember the taste in your mouth. What could you have done to change the outcome? Why didn't you do it then? What would you do if you had the chance to do it over?

Strength Training–Shoulders

ISO Front Raise–Isolateral (46): 10; 10; 10; 10

FW Lateral Raise–Dumbbell (26): 10; 10; 10; 10

FW High Pull–Dumbbell (24): 6; 6; 6; 6

FW Power Clean–Barbell (44): 5; 5; 5; 5

FW Shoulder Shrugs–Barbell (35): 10; 10; 10; 10

ISO Military Press–Isolateral (49): 8; 6; 6; 6

Abdominals

AB Roll-Ups (4): 15-20; 15-20; 15-20; 15-20

Cardiovascular Conditioning

CC Soft Sand or Grass Run (15a): 20-30 minutes
or
CC Treadmill Workout, Protocol C (20)

IW

Warm-Up

FE **Key's Catching Drills (84):** Choose 4 drills, 20 catches each way

AB **Good Mornings (2):** 10; 10; 10

CC **Jump Rope (13):** 60 seconds; 60 seconds; 60 seconds

Stretch

KSR Keyshawn Stretch Routine

Mental Training

Identify your dreams: What is your most outrageous dream? Identify the first step you could take toward making that dream a reality. Ask yourself what it would take to give you the courage to take that step.

Strength Training–Chest/Back/Legs

PL **Step-Ups (60):** 8 per leg; 8 per leg; 8 per leg; 8 per leg

PS **Squats–Medicine Ball or Plate (77):** 15; 15; 15

ME **Leg Extension (56):** 12; 12; 12

FW **Squats–Barbell (37):** 8; 8; 6; 6

FW **Pullovers–Dumbbell (30):** 8; 8; 6; 6

FW **Bench Press–Barbell (21):** 10; 8; 8; 6; 6

FW **Row–Dumbbell (34):** 8; 8; 6; 6

FW **Incline Press–Dumbbell (25):** 8; 8; 6; 6

Abdominals

AB **Bent Leg Crunch with Twist (6):** 20; 20; 20

AB **Decline Bench Medicine Ball Toss with Twist (9):** 30 seconds; 30 seconds; 30 seconds
or

AB **Good Mornings with Twist (3):** 6-8; 6-8; 6-8

Cardiovascular Conditioning

CC **Sprints (16):** 4 150-yard sprints, 6 100-yard sprints. Walk back to starting point.

CC **Steady Run or Jog (15b):** 5-8 minutes

Warm-Up

FW **Rice Grabs (33):** 45 seconds; 45 seconds; 45 seconds

PL **Step-Ups (60):** 30 seconds; 30 seconds; 30 seconds

Stretch

KSR **Keyshawn Stretch Routine**

Mental Training

Never forget who you are: What do you think your best characteristic is? Do other people see this part of you? If not, what can you do to make it more present in your life. If yes, what can you do to nurture it more?

Strength Training–Shoulders

FW **Front Raise–Dumbbell (23):** 10; 10; 10; 10

FW **Lateral Raise–Dumbbell (26):** 8; 8; 8; 8

FW **Push Press–Dumbbell (32):** 8; 8; 6; 6

FW **Shoulder Shrugs–Barbell (35):** 10; 10; 10; 10

FW **Upright Row–Barbell (41):** 8; 8; 6; 6

Abdominals

AB **V-Ups (5):** 15-18; 15-18; 15-18

AB **Roll-Ups (4):** 20-25; 20-25; 20-25

Cardiovascular Conditioning

CC **Soft Sand or Grass Run (15a)** *or* **Steady Run or Jog (15b):** 25-30 minutes
or
CC **Treadmill Workout, Protocol B (20)**

IW

Warm-Up

FW **Lunges—Body Weight (27):** 30 seconds; 30 seconds; 30 seconds

CC **Jump Rope (13):** 60 seconds; 60 seconds; 60 seconds

Stretch

KSR **Keyshawn Stretch Routine**

Mental Training

Develop a winning attitude: Visualize the reward you would receive or give yourself if you achieved a current goal.

Strength Training—Plyometrics

FE **V-Jumps (81):** 30 seconds; 30 seconds; 30 seconds

PS **In-Line Lateral Shuffle (71):** 20 seconds; 20 seconds; 20 seconds

PS **3-Cone Drill (67):** 20 seconds; 20 seconds; 20 seconds

PL **Box Jumps—Big Box (59b):** 6-8; 6-8; 6-8

PL **Medicine Ball Walk (63):** 15-20 yards; 15-20 yards; 15-20 yards

AB **Knee-Ups (12):** 40; 40; 40

Abdominals

AB **High Crunches (1):** 25; 25; 25

AB **Good Mornings (2):** 15; 15; 15

Cardiovascular Conditioning

CC **Sprints (16):** 10-12 sprints, 100 yards each. You have 60 seconds to sprint 100 yards and jog back to starting point.

Warm-Up

AB **Roll-Ups (4):** 12-15; 12-15; 12-15

AB **Good Mornings (2):** 12-15; 12-15; 12-15

Stretch

KSR Keyshawn Stretch Routine

Mental Training

Don't let others set your limits: Identify one way in which you are not achieving your potential because another person is in the way. What would it take to clear the path to your goal? Identify one step you can take toward this end.

Strength Training–Chest/Back/Legs

FW **Lunges–Dumbbell (28):** 20 reps per side; 20 reps per side; 20 reps per side

PL **Push-Ups–Plyometric (64):** 8-10; 8-10; 8-10

FW **Pull-Ups:** 8-10; 8-10; 8-10; 8-10

FW **Bench Press–Barbell (21):** 10; 8; 8; 6; 6

FW **Bench Press–Dumbbell (22):** 8; 8; 8

FW **Pullovers–Dumbbell (30):** 8; 8; 8; 8

FW **Incline Press–Dumbbell (25):** 8; 8; 6; 6

Abdominals

AB **V-Ups (5):** 15-20; 15-20; 15-20; 15-20

Cardiovascular Conditioning

CC **Treadmill Workout, Protocol C or D (20)**

CC **Steady Run or Jog (15b):** 5-8 minutes

IW

Warm-Up

FW **Rice Grabs (33):** 45 seconds; 45 seconds; 45 seconds

PL **Step-Ups (60):** 30 seconds; 30 seconds; 30 seconds

Stretch

KSR Keyshawn Stretch Routine

Mental Training

Do the best you can at one thing today!

Strength Training—Shoulders

FW **ISO** **Front Raise—Dumbell (23)** *or* **Isolateral (46):** 8; 8; 8; 8

FW **Lateral Raise—Dumbbell (26):** 8; 8; 8; 8

FW **Power Clean—Barbell (44):** 5; 5; 4; 4

FW **High Pull—Dumbbell (24):** 5; 5; 4; 4

FW **Military Press—Dumbbell (29):** 8; 8; 6; 6

FW **Upright Row—Barbell (41):** 8; 8; 6; 6

Abdominals

AB **High Crunches (1)** *or* **Decline Bench Medicine Ball Toss with Twist (9):** 20; 20; 20

AB **Good Mornings (2):** 15; 15; 15

Cardiovascular Conditioning

CC **Sprints (16):** 4 150-yard sprints, 6 100-yard sprints. Walk back to starting point.

CC **Steady Run or Jog (15b):** 5-8 minutes

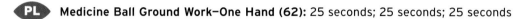
Warm-Up

PL Medicine Ball Ground Work–One Hand (62): 25 seconds; 25 seconds; 25 seconds

FW Lunges–Body Weight (27): 20 yards; 20 yards; 20 yards

Stretch

KSR Keyshawn Stretch Routine

Mental Training

Reflect on the experience of doing your best yesterday.

Strength Training–Chest/Back/Legs

PS Squats–Medicine Ball or Plate (77): 15; 15; 15

FW Squats–Barbell (37): 8; 8; 6; 6

ME Leg Extension (56): 10; 10; 10

ME Leg Flexion (57): 10; 10; 10

FW Bench Press–Barbell (21): 10; 8; 8; 6; 6

FW Row–Dumbbell (34): 8; 8; 6; 6

FW Incline Press–Dumbbell (25): 8; 8; 6; 6

FW Pull-Ups: 6-8; 6-8; 6-8

PS Medicine Ball Toss–Chest (74): 8-10; 8-10; 8-10

Abdominals

AB V-Ups (5): 12-14; 12-14 ; 12-14

AB Medicine Ball Plyometric Oblique Toss (10): 6-8; 6-8; 6-8

Cardiovascular Conditioning

CC Steady Run or Jog (15b): 25-30 minutes
or
CC Treadmill Workout, Protocol A (20)

Day 3

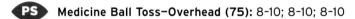

Warm-Up

PS Medicine Ball Toss–Overhead (75): 8-10; 8-10; 8-10

FW Lunges–Body Weight (27): 20 yards; 20 yards; 20 yards

Stretch

KSR Keyshawn Stretch Routine

Mental Training

Do your best at everything you do today!

Strength Training–Plyometrics

PL Lateral Jumps–Long Way (61): 20 seconds; 20 seconds; 20 seconds

PL Bench Squat with One Leg–Body Weight (65): 10; 10; 10; 10

FE Figure 8's (79): 30 seconds; 30 seconds; 30 seconds; 30 seconds

PL Box Jumps–Big Box (59b): 6-8; 6-8; 6-8

AB Knee-Ups (12): 40; 40; 40; 40

FE V-Jumps (81): 30 seconds; 30 seconds; 30 seconds

Abdominals

AB High Crunches (1): 25; 25; 25; 25

AB Good Mornings (2): 15; 15; 15; 15

Cardiovascular Conditioning

CC Sprints (16): 10-12 sprints, 100 yards each. You have 60 seconds to sprint 100 yards and jog back to starting point.

Warm-Up

AB Good Mornings (2): 15; 15; 15

FW Rice Grabs (33): 45 seconds; 45 seconds; 45 seconds

Stretch

KSR Keyshawn Stretch Routine

Mental Training

Reflect on the results of giving your best the whole day yesterday.

Strength Training–Legs and Shoulders

FW Straight-Leg Dead Lifts–Dumbbell (40): 10; 10; 10; 10

FW Squats–Dumbbell (38): 10; 10; 8; 8

FW Shoulder Shrugs–Dumbbell (36): 10; 10; 10; 10

FW Lateral Raise–Dumbbell (26): 8; 8; 8; 8

FW Push Press–Dumbbell (32): 8; 8; 6; 6

FW Power Clean–Barbell (44): 5; 5; 4; 4

FW Upright Row–Barbell (41): 8; 8; 6; 6

Abdominals

AB V-Ups (5): 15-20; 15-20; 15-20; 15-20

Cardiovascular Conditioning

CC Explosive Running (19): 8-10 reps, 40 yards each, 30-second rest between reps

CC Steady Run or Jog (15b): 5-8 minutes

IW

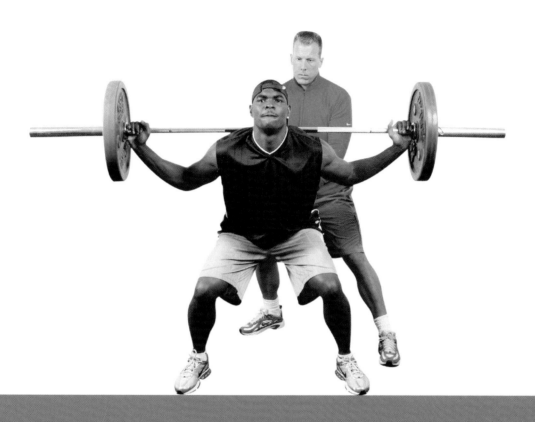

Advanced Workout–4 to 5 days/week

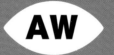

The advanced workout should be six weeks long. Start the workout with the two-week routine described here, then go back to the intermediate workout, using the routine described there but adding an exercise to each day from the strength training group of that day. For example, if the strength training is focused on plyometrics that day, add another plyometric exercise; if it is focused on legs, add a leg exercise. Use the number of reps and sets that is given for the exercise (or for similar exercises) elsewhere in the intermediate routine.

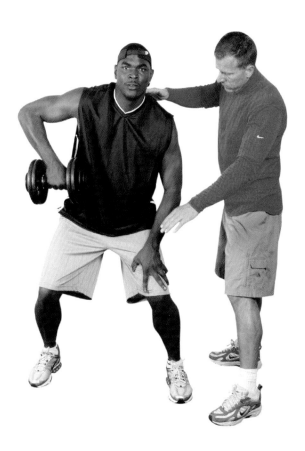

Warm-Up

AB **V-Ups (5):** 10-12; 10-12; 10-12

FE **Key's Catching Drills (84):** Choose 4 drills, 20 catches each way

Stretch

KSR **Keyshawn Stretch Routine**

Mental Training

Believe in yourself: Remember a time when standing your ground caused you to succeed. Examine the event carefully, remembering the feeling of believing in your opinion and succeeding.

Strength Training–Shoulders

FW **Curls–Dumbbell (42):** 10; 10; 10; 10

FW **Front Raise–Dumbbell (23):** 10; 10; 10; 10

FW **High Pull–Dumbbell (24):** 6; 6; 6; 6

FW **Power Clean–Barbell (44):** 5; 5; 5; 5

FW **Shoulder Shrugs–Barbell (35):** 10; 10; 10; 10

FW **Military Press–Dumbbell (29):** 8; 6; 6; 6

Abdominals

AB **Roll-Ups (4):** 15-20; 15-20; 15-20; 15-20

Cardiovascular Conditioning

CC **Soft Sand or Grass Run (15a):** 20-30 minutes

FE **Bounce and Catch (85):** 6; 6; 6

PS **In-Line Knee-Ups (72):** 4 sets, 1 minute 30 seconds between sets

AW

Day 2

Warm-Up

PS **4-Cone Drill (68):** 3 sets, 60-second rest between sets

AB **Good Mornings (2):** 10; 10; 10

CC **Jump Rope (13):** 60 seconds; 60 seconds; 60 seconds

Stretch

KSR **Keyshawn Stretch Routine**

Mental Training

Put worry where it belongs: Identify something you are concerned about. Are you exerting energy in worrying about it? If yes, identify one step you can take to improve the situation and redirect your energy toward that end.

Strength Training—Legs/Chest/Back

PL **Step-Ups (60):** 8 per leg; 8 per leg; 8 per leg; 8 per leg

PS **Squats–Medicine Ball or Plate (77):** 15; 15; 15

FW **Squats–Barbell (37):** 8; 8; 6; 6
or
ME **Leg Press (58):** 10; 10; 10; 10

ME **Leg Extension (56):** 10; 10; 8; 8

ME **Leg Flexion (57):** 10; 10; 8; 8

ME **Pull-Downs–Reverse Grip (55):** 8; 8; 8

FW **Pullovers–Dumbbell (30):** 8; 8; 6; 6

FW **Bench Press–Barbell (21):** 10; 8; 8; 6; 6

FW **Row–Dumbbell (34):** 8; 8; 6; 6

FW **Incline Press–Dumbbell (25):** 8; 8; 6; 6

Abdominals

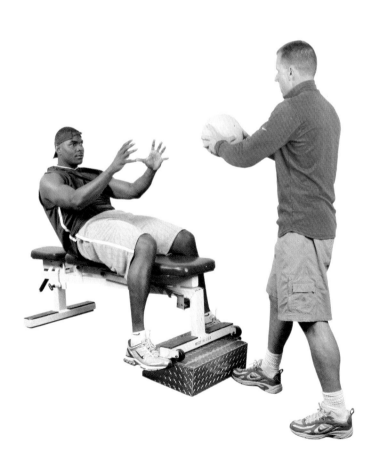

AB Medicine Ball Plyometric Oblique Toss (10): 12-14; 12-14; 12-14

AB Decline Bench Crunch with Medicine Ball (7): 15; 15; 15

Cardiovascular Conditioning

CC Sprints (16): 4 150-yard sprints, 6 100-yard sprints. Walk back to starting point.

CC Steady Run or Jog (15b): 5-8 minutes

PS 3-Cone Drill (67): 3 sets of 3 reps

FE Diagonal Shuffle (80): 3 sets of 3 reps

AW

Day 3

Warm-Up

FW **Rice Grabs (33):** 45 seconds; 45 seconds; 45 seconds

PL **Step-Ups (60):** 30 seconds; 30 seconds; 30 seconds

Stretch

KSR **Keyshawn Stretch Routine**

Mental Training

Create success: Call to mind your picture of yourself when you began working out. Compare this picture with the one you have of yourself today. In what ways have you improved? What is left to be done?

Strength Training–Shoulders

FW **Front Raise–Dumbbell (23):** 10; 10; 10; 10

FW **Lateral Raise–Dumbbell (26):** 8; 8; 8; 8

FW **Push Press–Dumbbell (32):** 8; 8; 6; 6

FW **Shoulder Shrugs–Barbell (35):** 10; 10; 10; 10

FW **Upright Row–Barbell (41):** 8; 8; 6; 6

FW **Power Clean–Barbell (44):** 5; 5; 4; 4

Abdominals

AB **V-Ups (5):** 15-18; 15-18; 15-18

AB **Roll-Ups (4):** 20-25; 20-25; 20-25

Cardiovascular Conditioning

CC **Soft Sand or Grass Run (15a):** 25-30 minutes
or
CC **Treadmill Workout, Protocol B** *or* **D (20)**

FE **Pick 3 drills from Fieldwork Exercises.** Complete 3 sets of 3 reps each for each drill.

Warm-Up

FE Key's Catching Drills (84): Choose 4 drills, 20 catches each way

CC Jump Rope (13): 60 seconds; 60 seconds; 60 seconds

Stretch

KSR Keyshawn Stretch Routine

Mental Training

Seek inspiration: Identify one of your heroes. What is it about this person that attracts you? Do you share any of the same characteristics? Identify one specific thing that your hero inspires you to attempt. Put that inspiration into action!

Strength Training–Plyometrics

PL Push-Ups–Plyometric (64): 8-10; 8-10; 8-10

FE V-Jumps (81): 30 seconds; 30 seconds; 30 seconds

PL Bench Squat with One Leg–Body Weight (65): 10; 10; 10; 10

PL Box Jumps–Big Box (59b): 6-8; 6-8; 6-8

PS Medicine Ball Toss–Overhead (75): 6; 6; 6; 6

AB Knee-Ups (12): 40; 40; 40

Abdominals

AB High Crunches (1): 25; 25; 25

AB Good Mornings (2): 15; 15; 15

Cardiovascular Conditioning

CC Sprints (16): 10-12 sprints, 100 yards each. You have 60 seconds to sprint 100 yards and jog back to starting point.

CC Resistance Running (18): 20 yards; 20 yards; 20 yards; 20 yards; 20 yards

FE Diagonal Shuffle (80): 4 sets, 3 reps each, 30-second rest between sets

AW

Warm-Up

PS **3-Way Warm-Up (66):** 3 sets of 3 reps each

AB **Good Mornings (2):** 12-15; 12-15; 12-15

Stretch

KSR Keyshawn Stretch Routine

Mental Training

Don't settle for less than you can be: As an athlete, what is your greatest weakness? Identify the strategies you have used so far to improve in this area. Why haven't they worked? Identify one new tactic you could take to improve and work it into today's workout.

Strength Training-Legs/Chest/Back

FW **Lunges—Dumbbell (28):** 20 reps per side; 20 reps per side; 20 reps per side; 20 reps per side

PL **Push-Ups—Plyometric (64):** 8-10; 8-10; 8-10; 8-10

ME **Leg Extension (56):** 10; 10; 8; 8

ME **Leg Flexion (57):** 10; 10; 8; 8

FW **Pull-Ups:** 8-10; 8-10; 8-10; 8-10

FW **Bench Press—Barbell (21):** 10; 8; 8; 6; 6

FW **Pullovers—Dumbbell (30):** 8; 8; 8; 8

FW **Incline Press—Dumbbell (25):** 8; 8; 6; 6

Abdominals

AB **V-Ups (5):** 15-20; 15-20; 15-20; 15-20

AB **Bent Leg Crunch with Twist (6):** 15; 15; 15; 15

Cardiovascular Conditioning

CC **Run and Hold (17):** 10 sets. Run 20 yards and hold for 10 seconds. Your rest period should be 1 minute to 1 minute 20 seconds.

CC **Steady Run or Jog (15b):** 5-8 minutes

Warm-Up

FW **Rice Grabs (33):** 45 seconds; 45 seconds; 45 seconds

PL **Step-Ups (60):** 30 seconds; 30 seconds; 30 seconds

Stretch

KSR **Keyshawn Stretch Routine**

Mental Training

Never forget who you are: What did friends from your youth say your best characteristic was? Do you still have that quality? What has it allowed you to achieve? What could you achieve if you were to focus on it more clearly?

Strength Training–Shoulders

ISO **Front Raise–Isolateral (46):** 8; 8; 8; 8

FW **Lateral Raise–Dumbbell (26):** 8; 8; 8; 8

FW **Military Press–Dumbbell (29):** 5; 5; 4; 4

FW **High Pull–Dumbbell (24):** 5; 5; 4; 4

FW **Push Press–Dumbbell (32):** 8; 8; 6; 6

FW **Upright Row–Barbell (41):** 8; 8; 6; 6

FW **Power Clean–Barbell (44):** 4; 4; 3; 3

Abdominals

AB **Roll-Ups (4):** 20; 20; 20; 20

AB **Leg Throws (11):** 15; 15; 15; 15

Cardiovascular Conditioning

CC **Sprints (16):** 4 150-yard sprints, 6 100-yard sprints. Walk back to starting point.

CC **Steady Run or Jog (15b):** 5-8 minutes
or
CC **Treadmill Workout, Protocol B or D (20)**

FE **Pick 3 drills from Fieldwork Exercises.** For each drill, complete 3 sets of 3 reps each.

AW

Day 2

Warm-Up

PL **Medicine Ball Ground Work–One Hand (62):** 20 yards; 20 yards; 20 yards

FW **Lunges–Body Weight (27):** 20 yards; 20 yards; 20 yards

FE **Key's Catching Drills (84):** Choose 2 drills, 20 catches each way

Stretch

KSR **Keyshawn Stretch Routine**

Mental Training

Demand a lot from yourself: Identify the part of today's workout that you are inclined to take easily. Don't. Challenge yourself to do your very best in that area.

Strength Training–Legs/Chest/Back

PS **Squats–Medicine Ball or Plate (77):** 15; 15; 15

FW **Squats–Dumbbell (38):** 8; 8; 6; 6; 6
or
ME **Leg Press (58):** 10; 10; 8; 8

FW **Bench Press–Barbell (21):** 10; 8; 8; 6; 6

ME **Leg Extension (56):** 8; 8; 8; 8

ME **Leg Flexion (57):** 8; 8; 8; 8

FW **Row–Dumbbell (34):** 8; 8; 6; 6

FW **Incline Press–Dumbbell (25):** 8; 8; 6; 6

FW **Pull-Ups:** 6-8; 6-8; 6-8

PS **Medicine Ball Toss–Chest (74):** 8-10; 8-10; 8-10

Abdominals

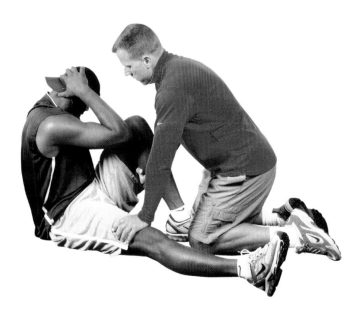

AB **Bent Leg Crunch with Twist (6):** 25; 25; 25

AB **Roll-Ups (4):** 20; 20; 20

Cardiovascular Conditioning

CC **Soft Sand or Grass Run (15a):** 25-30 minutes

FE **Pick 3 drills from Fieldwork Exercises.** For each drill, complete 3 sets of 3 reps each.

AW

Warm-Up

PS Medicine Ball Toss—Overhead (75): 8-10; 8-10; 8-10

FW Lunges—Body Weight (27): 30 seconds; 30 seconds; 30 seconds

Stretch

KSR Keyshawn Stretch Routine

Mental Training

Determine to do your best in every part of your workout today.

Strength Training—Plyometrics

PL Lateral Jumps—Long Way (61): 30 seconds; 30 seconds; 30 seconds

FE In-Line Vertical Jumps (82): 3 sets of 3 reps

FE Diagonal Shuffle (80): 30 seconds; 30 seconds; 30 seconds; 30 seconds

PL Box Jumps—Big Box (59b): 8; 8; 8; 8

AB Knee-Ups (12): 40; 40; 40; 40

FE V-Jumps (81): 30 seconds; 30 seconds; 30 seconds

Abdominals

AB High Crunches (1): 25; 25; 25; 25

AB Good Mornings (2): 15; 15; 15; 15

Cardiovascular Conditioning

CC Sprints (16): 10-12 sprints, 100 yards each. You have 60 seconds to sprint 100 yards and jog back to starting point.
or

CC Treadmill Workout, Protocol C (20)

Warm-Up

AB **Roll-Ups (4):** 20; 20; 20

FW **Rice Grabs (33):** 45 seconds; 45 seconds; 45 seconds

Stretch

KSR Keyshawn Stretch Routine

Mental Training

Determine to do your best at everything you do today.

Strength Training—Legs and Shoulders

FW **Straight-Leg Dead Lifts—Barbell (39):** 10; 10; 10; 10

FW **Squats—Dumbbell (38):** 10; 10; 8; 8

FW **Shoulder Shrugs—Dumbbell (36):** 10; 10; 10; 10

FW **Lateral Raise—Dumbbell (26):** 8; 8; 8; 8

FW **Push Press—Dumbbell (32):** 8; 8; 6; 6

FW **Power Clean—Barbell (44):** 5; 5; 4; 4

FW **Upright Row—Barbell (41):** 8; 8; 6; 6

Abdominals

AB **V-Ups (5):** 15-20; 15-20; 15-20; 15-20

Cardiovascular Conditioning

CC **Run and Hold (17):** 10 sets. Run 20 yards and hold for 10 seconds. Your rest period should be 1 minute to 1 minute 20 seconds.
or

CC **Resistance Running (18):** 5 reps, 3 sets of 20 yards

CC **Steady Run or Jog (15b):** 5-8 minutes

AW

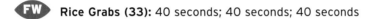

Warm-Up

FW **Rice Grabs (33):** 40 seconds; 40 seconds; 40 seconds

CC **Jump Rope (13):** 60 seconds; 60 seconds; 60 seconds

Stretch

KSR Keyshawn Stretch Routine

Mental Training

Reflect on the experience of doing your best at everything yesterday.

Strength Training–Plyometrics

FE **In-Line Vertical Jumps (82):** 30 seconds; 30 seconds; 30 seconds; 30 seconds

PS **In-Line Lateral Shuffle (71):** 30 seconds; 30 seconds; 30 seconds

PS **In-Line Knee-Ups (72):** 30 seconds; 30 seconds; 30 seconds; 30 seconds

PL **Box Jumps–Big Box (59b):** 6-8; 6-8; 6-8

PL **Medicine Ball Ground Work–One Hand (62):** 30 seconds; 30 seconds; 30 seconds; 30 seconds

AB **Knee-Ups (12):** 40; 40; 40

Abdominals

AB **High Crunches (1):** 25; 25; 25

AB **Good Mornings (2):** 15; 15; 15

Cardiovascular Conditioning

CC **Sprints (16):** 10-12 sprints, 100 yards each. You have 60 seconds to sprint 100 yards and jog back to starting point.

FE **Pick 3 drills from Fieldwork Exercises.** For each drill, complete 4 sets of 3 reps each.

Notes

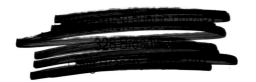

Notes